AF786635

Recent Results in Cancer Research 78

Fortschritte der Krebsforschung
Progrès dans les recherches sur le cancer

Edited by

V. G. Allfrey, New York · M. Allgöwer, Basel
I. Berenblum, Rehovot · F. Bergel, Jersey
J. Bernard, Paris · W. Bernhard, Villejuif
N. N. Blokhin, Moskva · H. E. Bock, Tübingen
W. Braun, New Brunswick · P. Bucalossi, Milano
A. V. Chaklin, Moskva · M. Chorazy, Gliwice
G. J. Cunningham, Richmond · G. Della Porta, Milano
P. Denoix, Villejuif · R. Dulbecco, La Jolla
H. Eagle, New York · R. Eker, Oslo
R. A. Good, New York · P. Grabar, Paris
R. J. C. Harris, Salisbury · E. Hecker, Heidelberg
R. Herbeuval, Vandoeuvre · J. Higginson, Lyon
W. C. Hueper, Fort Myers · H. Isliker, Lausanne
J. Kieler, Kobenhavn · W. H. Kirsten, Chicago
G. Klein, Stockholm · H. Koprowski, Philadelphia
L. G. Koss, New York · R. A. Macbeth, Toronto
G. Martz, Zürich · G. Mathé, Villejuif
O. Mühlbock, Amsterdam · L. J. Old, New York
V. R. Potter, Madison · A. B. Sabin, Charleston, S.C.
L. Sachs, Rehovot · E. A. Saxén, Helsinki
C. G. Schmidt, Essen · S. Spiegelman, New York
W. Szybalski, Madison · H. Tagnon, Bruxelles
A. Tissières, Genève · E. Uehlinger, Zürich
R. W. Wissler, Chicago

Editor in Chief: P. Rentchnick, Genève
Co-editor: H. J. Senn, St. Gallen

Recent Results 78

H. J. Senn, St. Gallen

Prostate Cancer

Edited by William Duncan

With 68 Figures and 67 Tables

Springer-Verlag
Berlin Heidelberg New York 1981

Professor William Duncan

Department of Radiation Oncology
Western General Hospital and
Royal Infirmary, Grewe Road
Edinburgh EH4 2XU, United Kingdom

Sponsored by the Swiss League against Cancer

ISBN-13: 978-3-642-81623-9 e-ISBN-13: 978-3-642-81621-5
DOI: 10.1007/978-3-642-81621-5

Library of Congress Cataloging in Publication Data. Main entry under title: Prostate cancer. (Recent results in cancer research; 78) Based on papers presented at the Second Symposium on Clinical Oncology held by the Royal College of Radiologists, February 1980 in London and sponsored by the Swiss League against Cancer. Bibliography: p. Includes index. Contents: Epidemiology / M. R. Alderson – Morphology in health and disease / N. J. Blacklock – Growth kinetics / M. R. Alison and N. A. Wright – [etc.] 1. Prostate gland – Cancer – Congresses. I. Duncan, William, 1930 –. II. Symposium on Clinical Oncology (2nd : 1980 : London) III. Royal College of Radiologists (Great Britain) IV. Schweizerische Nationalliga für Krebsbekämpfung und Krebsforschung. V. Series. [DNLM: 1. Prostate neoplasms – Congresses. W1 RE106P v. 78 / WJ 752 P9654 1980] RC261.R35 vol. 78 [RC280.P7] 616.99'4s 81-2643 [616.99'463] AACR2

This work is subject to copyright. All rights are reserved, whether the whole or part of the material is concerned, specifically those of translation, reprinting, re-use of illustrations, broadcasting, reproduction by photocopying machine or similar means, and storage in data banks. Under § 54 of the German Copyright Law where copies are made for other than private use a fee is payable to 'Verwertungsgesellschaft Wort', Munich.

© Springer-Verlag Berlin Heidelberg 1981

Softcover reprint of the hardcover 1st edition 1981

The use of registered names, trademarks, etc. in the publication does not imply, even in the absence of a specific statement, that such names are exempt from the relevant protective laws and regulations and therefore free for general use.

2125/3140–543210

Preface

In February 1980 the Royal College of Radiologists, London, held its Second Symposium on Clinical Oncology. The subject was Prostatic Cancer and this publication is based on the presentations at this meeting by leading authorities in the United Kingdom.

The principal objective of these Symposia is to promote multidisciplinary collaboration for the benefit of cancer patients. Awareness and understanding of advances in a broad range of subjects are essential to ensure the timely and effective application of new techniques in the prevention and treatment of all forms of cancer. Communication of this kind may also stimulate the creation of new ideas that may prove to be of more fundamental relevance to cancer research.

Prostatic cancer has been afforded too little attention in the past, and its importance in Clinical Oncology has not been adequately recognised. And yet over the last 10 years considerable progress has been recorded in our understanding of this disease and in its assessment and management. These achievements are well documented in this collection of papers and the outstanding problems are also clearly indicated. It is acknowledged that the early diagnosis of prostatic cancer presents a continuing challenge, associated with the uncertainties that concern the clinical significance of 'latent' cancer of the prostate. The accurate assessment of the incidence and prevalence of the disease is extremely difficult and together these problems complicate the evaluation of the management of early or localised prostatic cancer.

There have been major developments in epidemiological, laboratory, and clinical research into prostatic cancer. There is now much better understanding of the form and function of the prostate and of its control. Considerable technical progress has been made in the assay of steroid receptors and in the refinement of tumour marker assay. Methods of imaging the prostate have greatly improved and nuclear medicine, particularly in the role of bone scintigraphy, is recognised to be of prime importance in the assessment of patients with prostatic cancer. Another great change in the last decade has been the increasing use of radiotherapy in the primary management of patients with localised carcinoma of the prostate. Excellent long-term disease-free survival rates have been reported, and much more optimistic attitudes to the treatment of this disease have resulted. The administration of oestrogens is now advised for much more limited clinical indications following a series of extremely well-designed and carefully conducted clinical trials; their routine use for localised cancer of the prostate can no longer be regarded as an acceptable policy.

These developments are well reviewed in this volume and it is to be hoped that its publication may stimulate further interest in this fascinating disease. I have to express my gratitude to those who took part in the Symposium and also to their colleagues who have contributed to the texts for publication. I have also to record my appreciation to Mr. Michael Jackson of Springer-Verlag for his advice and understanding, and to his editorial staff who have helped to ensure prompt publication. My thanks are also extended to my personal secretary Mrs. Joyce Young, who ably assisted in the organisation of the Symposium as well as in the preparation of the scripts for publication.

Royal College of Radiologists, London WILLIAM DUNCAN

Contents

M. R. Alderson:
Epidemiology 1

N. J. Blacklock:
Morphology in Health and Disease 20

M. R. Alison and N. A. Wright:
Growth Kinetics 29

M. E. Harper, P. Chaisiri, J. Slade, W. B. Peeling, and K. Griffiths:
Hormonal Relationships, Receptors, and Tumour Markers 44

R. C. B. Pugh:
Pathology and Natural History 60

H. Mamtora, M. R. Gowland, and I. Isherwood:
Diagnostic Imaging 76

J. S. Macdonald:
Lymphography 97

M. V. Merrick, A. R. Stone, and G. D. Chisholm:
Nuclear Medicine 108

W. F. Hendry:
Surgery 119

H. J. G. Bloom:
Radiotherapy 132

P. H. Smith:
Endocrine and Cytotoxic Therapy 154

G. D. Chisholm:
Perspectives and Prospects 173

Subject Index 185

List of Senior Authors

M. R. Alderson
Department of Epidemiology, Institute of Cancer Research, London, United Kingdom

M. R. Alison
Department of Histopathology, Royal Postgraduate Medical School, London, United Kingdom

N. J. Blacklock
Department of Urology, University of Manchester, Manchester, United Kingdom

H. J. G. Bloom
Department of Radiotherapy and Oncology, Royal Marsden Hospital and Institute of Cancer Research, London, United Kingdom

G. D. Chisholm
Department of Surgery (Urology), University of Edinburgh, Edinburgh, United Kingdom

P. Chaisiri
Tenovus Institute for Cancer Research, The Welsh National School of Medicine, Cardiff, United Kingdom

M. R. Gowland
Department of Diagnostic Radiology, University of Manchester, Manchester, United Kingdom

K. Griffiths
Tenovus Institute for Cancer Research, The Welsh National School of Medicine, Cardiff, United Kingdom

M. E. Harper
Tenovus Institute for Cancer Research, The Welsh National School of Medicine, Cardiff, United Kingdom

W. F. Hendry
St. Bartholomews and Royal Marsden Hospital and Institute of Urology, London, United Kingdom

I. Isherwood
Department of Diagnostic Radiology, University of Manchester, Manchester, United Kingdom

J. S. Macdonald
Department of Diagnostic Radiology, Royal Marsden Hospital, and Institute of Cancer Research, London, United Kingdom

H. Mantora
Department of Diagnostic Radiology, University of Manchester, Manchester, United Kingdom

M. V. Merrick
Department of Surgery (Urology), University of Edinburgh, Edinburgh, United Kingdom

W. B. Peeling
Tenovus Institute for Cancer Research, The Welsh National School of Medicine, Cardiff, United Kingdom

R. C. B. Pugh
Department of Pathology, Institute of Urology, London, United Kingdom

J. Slade
Tenovus Institute for Cancer Research, The Welsh National School of Medicine, Cardiff, United Kingdom

P. H. Smith
Department of Urology, St. James's University Hospital, Leeds, United Kingdom

A. R. Stone
Department of Surgery (Urology), University of Edinburgh, Edinburgh, United Kingdom

N. A. Wright
Department of Histopathology, Royal Postgraduate Medical School, London, United Kingdom

Epidemiology

M. R. Alderson*

Department of Epidemiology, Institute of Cancer Research, GB – London

1 Introduction

This chapter reviews present knowledge of the aetiology of prostate cancer. Routine mortality and incidence statistics are examined both for England and Wales and for other countries, as are the results of a range of special studies. The chapter begins with a brief note on the problem of the diagnosis of prostate cancer, and its import as far as the validity of routine statistics is concerned. The review of aetiological studies does not result in any clear pointers to factors that could be avoided to achieve any marked effect on the incidence of this condition. Because of the relatively high toll of the disease it is important to consider whether any steps can be taken to reduce the delay prior to diagnosis and treatment. The chapter therefore ends with a brief consideration of the value of screening for this disease.

2 Validity of Routine Statistics

2.1 What is Prostate Cancer?

Morgagni (1760) demonstrated that suppression of urine could be caused by "preternatural swelling of the prostate gland"; he mentioned the type, social standing, and life habits of the patients. He was presumably referring to benign prostate hyperplasia, but it is worth considering the long history of concern about abnormalities of the prostate gland. Riches (1958) drew attention to the importance of the prostate as a site of malignant disease and suggested that it occurred in three rather different forms: latent, occult (with widespread metastases), and local definitive cancer. Rich (1935) reported 292 consecutive autopsies on males 50 years old and more; routine microscopical section identified 41 cases (14.0%) with frank carcinoma of the prostate, two-thirds of which were not recognised clinically. Edwards et al. (1953) examined sections of prostates from 173 consecutive autopsies in males 40 years and older, and 16.7% of the subjects were found to have a latent cancer of the prostate. Franks (1954) emphasised that latent cancer of the prostate was common and that its incidence increased with age; he suggested that the tumour has both morphological and

* Financial support of the Division of Epidemiology by the Cancer Research Campaign is gratefully acknowledged. I also thank Mrs. D. Folkes for preparing the text and Mrs. C. Beaven for the statistics and art work

Recent Results in Cancer Research, Vol. 78
© Springer-Verlag Berlin · Heidelberg 1981

biological characteristics of true malignancy, but lacks the capacity for rapid growth. In another contribution (Franks 1956) it was suggested that after the age of 80 the disease becomes common and over 90 years of age almost all men have these lesions (no hard data supporting this comment were provided). In an extensive study by Halpert et al. (1963) the prevalence increased with each successive decade of age. Scott et al. (1969) carried out step section at 4-mm intervals throughout the entire prostate for each of 158 males dying aged 70 and over. In 48% prostatic cancer was identified; this was twice the prevalence usually found at routine autopsy. The International Agency for Research in Cancer (Breslow et al. 1977) coordinated a study in which 50 prostates were collected from consecutive male autopsies in the age groups 45–, 55–, 65–, and 75+ from seven locations throughout the world. Duplicate readings were made by two pathologists in each case; and an exchange of opinions reduced the number of major differences in histological reporting. The frequency of small latent carcinoma was about 12% in all geographic areas involved. The distribution of larger latent carcinoma resembled that of clinical cancer, with a low frequency of latent carcinoma in two Chinese populations, an intermediate rate in Israelis and black Ugandans, and a high rate for German, Swedish, and black Jamaican populations. These findings agreed with those recorded in the more restricted groups studied in Japan (Karube 1961) and Hawaii (Akazaki and Stemmerman 1973).

Montgomery et al. (1961) followed up a small group of 35 patients with latent cancer of the prostate; after an average of nearly 7 years 24 of the subjects had died, but not one from prostate cancer. They suggest that specific treatment is not necessarily required when latent cancer is identified.

2.2 Some General Caveats

Mortality and routine incidence data are subject to a variety of errors and biases (see Alderson 1977). The mortality statistics are derived from death certificates stating that the prostate cancer was the underlying cause of death. Latent cancer, even if it has been diagnosed, will not be reflected in published mortality statistics if it does not contribute to the cause of death. If overt cancer is present, but the individual is thought to have died from some other disease, cancer may be mentioned on the certificate; at present multiple cause coding is not routinely published, and therefore one cannot tabulate statistics on the numbers of individuals having prostate cancer at the time of death.

The validity of the incidence data is rather different: whether the cancer is latent, occult, or overt, if it is recognised at some stage of the patient's treatment as being present it can be registered and reflected in the statistics. However, most probably only those prostate cancers investigated (and perhaps treated) are likely to be included in the registration statistics.

3 Mortality and Incidence Data

3.1 England and Wales

Figure 1 shows the age-specific mortality for England and Wales for 1973 and the incidence rates for 1970. The data are plotted on semi-log paper, and show a very steep

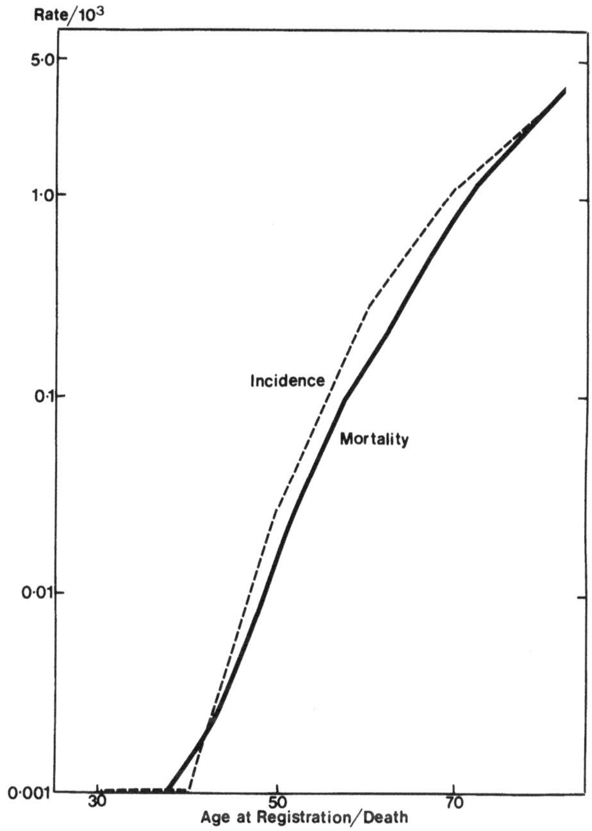

Fig. 1. Malignant neoplasm of prostate incidence rates, 1970, and mortality rates, 1973, by age at registration or death, England and Wales

rise in both incidence and mortality with advancing age. The other point to note is that the relative excess of incidence over mortality is very slight, indicating either that only a small proportion of subjects developing the disease are cured, or that the two sets of data are not equally valid. The excess mortality in the younger age groups is probably a reflection of small numbers, aggregation by age group, and differences in validity of the data.

Another way of looking at the age effect of this disease is to examine the cumulative frequency of distribution of deaths by age; such material is presented in Fig. 2 for England and Wales for the period 1971–1975. This shows how very few of the deaths occur in individuals under the age of 60, and that less than half the cases occur under the age of about 75.

Figure 3 shows the trends in mortality and incidence during the present century; five specific age groups have been selected, to reduce the number of lines on the graph. Data on mortality are available from 1911, but on incidence only since 1961. At the younger ages (i.e., up to 55–59) the mortality has not appreciably altered this century. For males aged 65–69 the mortality increased up until the 1930s but has since been relatively stable, whilst the mortality in males aged 75–79 increased fairly steadily up until about 1960 before levelling off. The incidence data are plotted for 10-year age groups and they are only available over a 13-year span (1961–1973). For the two older age groups there is a suggestion that the incidence is rising in the most recent material. Examination of these data plotted in different ways suggests that at least a proportion

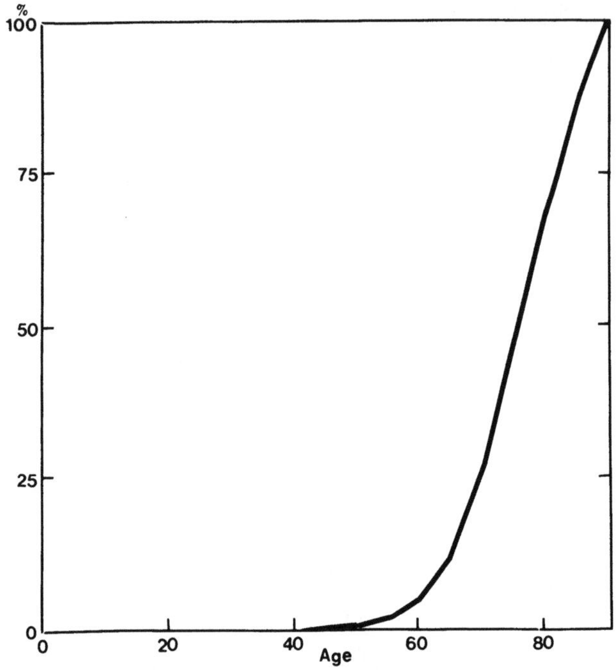

Fig. 2. Cumulative frequency distribution of deaths from malignant neoplasm of prostate in 1971–1975 by age, England and Wales

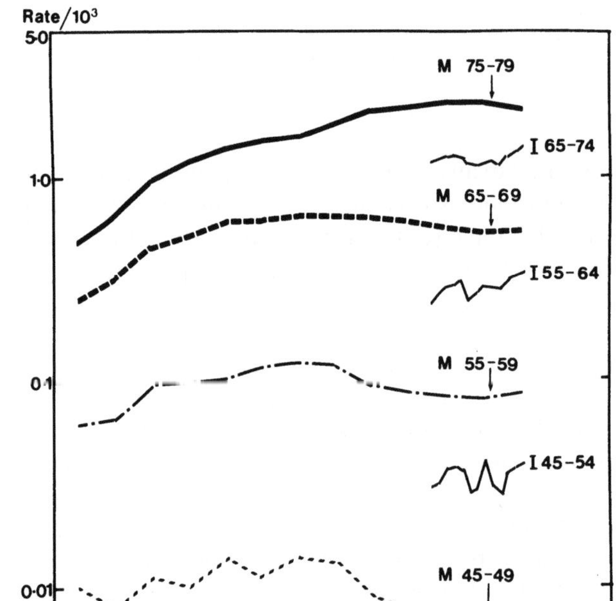

Fig. 3. Age-specific mortality rates for malignant neoplasm of prostate for 1911–1975 (*M*) and incidence rates for 1961–1973 (*I*), by year of registration or death, England and Wales

of the rise in the elderly is attributable to diagnostic factors rather than a general environmental factor or any difference in behaviour from one cohort to another.

3.2 International

In an attempt to examine the international variation in this disease and also any association with a cancer that is typical of 'Western' society, the age-specific mortality for cancer of the prostate against cancer of the lung was examined for 50 countries around 1976. There is considerable variation in the mortality rates for both conditions, with no suggestion of a relationship between the two. Even if an environmental factor is responsible for prostate cancer it has not spread in different countries in parallel with the development of smoking.

Other work has suggested a relationship between prostate cancer and sexual activity, and perhaps multiple consorts or acquisition of venereal disease (see Sect. 6). Data have been examined for cancer of the prostate and cancer of the cervix; unfortunately, however, the published mortality statistics for cancer of the cervix show that the proportion of cases ascribed to cervix cancer (compared with unspecified uterus cancer) varies markedly from one country to another. Both Hill (1975) and Weiss (1978) drew attention to the major problem in interpreting uterine cancer mortality, namely that cancer of the body of the uterus is frequently misclassified. Consideration of these points leads to the conclusion that it would be inappropriate to use national mortality statistics to seek a possible relationship between levels of cervix and prostate cancer.

Lancaster (1952) commented upon the increase in the death rate related to specifically male cancers in Australia over a relatively short period of time. Over the same time period there was no evident increase in the mortality from prostate hyperplasia and therefore no evidence that the increased incidence of cancer had been due to a shift in diagnosis. Ravich (1978) suggested that calculation of the incidence of this condition in Japan was unreliable; he ignored the method by which population incidence rates are normally calculated and compared.

Henschke et al. (1973) reviewed the mortality trends in the United States for 58 sites of cancer for whites and non-whites by sex, in the period 1950–1967. Prostate cancer was included in the group which had 'increased' significantly more slowly in the whites than blacks. After consideration of a number of defects in the data they suggested that 'environment' may be the main influence.

Ernster et al. (1978a) examined the cohort mortality for prostatic cancer amongst United States whites and non-whites. They showed a quite clear cohort mortality trend in the non-whites (but not for the whites). There were increasing rates of mortality in the cohorts born in 1846–1896 and then a complete reversal in the trend, with a decrease in age-specific mortality in the cohorts born after 1900. They concluded that alteration in medical care, screening, or accuracy of diagnosis is unlikely to have caused this picture, and that an aetiological factor had altered its impact on the non-whites in the United States in the groups born up to the beginning of the present century.

Jackson et al. (1975) report preliminary findings from a collaborative study in which data have been collected from patients with prostate cancer in the United States and Nigeria. They suggested that (i) the cancer is common in both United States and Nigerian blacks, and (ii) the Nigerian patients had less well-differentiated tumours, with more numerous foci of cancer, and lesions that were at a later stage of presentation.

Tulinius (1977) examined the incidence and mortality from prostate cancer in data collected from a large number of countries (45 countries for mortality). He drew attention to the very sharp increase in the incidence of and mortality from this condition in the elderly and very elderly (in contrast to other cancers); he pointed out that as the proportion of elderly persons in any population rises there will be a particularly marked increase in the total number of prostate cancer patients.

4 Genetic Factors

Lynch et al. (1966) reported a family of seven siblings, five of whom developed histologically proven cancer. Three brothers had carcinoma of the prostate, and two of these had other primary cancers as well. These findings were compared with the material from 109 consecutive patients treated with cancer of the prostate; for only five of these (4.5%) was a first-degree relative with the same cancer reported.

An estimate of the rarity of family aggregations cannot readily be made from such reports.

Woolf (1960) traced the death certificates for parents and siblings of 228 subjects dying from carcinoma of the prostate; he compared the causes of death of the relatives with those of control subjects. Death from prostate cancer was about three times as frequent in the relatives of the index patients as in the controls ($p < 0.05$). Three case-control studies, examining a range of factors, found an excess of positive family histories in the prostate cancer cases (Steele et al. 1971; Krain 1974; Schumann et al. 1977). Thiessen (1974) compared the family histories of 145 women with breast cancer against results from age-matched controls. A significant excess of prostatic cancer (and also breast and uterus cancer) was reported in both maternal and paternal relatives.

4.1 Blood Group

Bourke and Griffin (1962) compared the blood group distribution of 224 prostate cancer patients with that of 10,000 controls; they found a significant excess of blood group A in the cancer patients, and those with blood group A were younger at diagnosis. No difference was found between subjects with benign prostatic hypertrophy and controls. Wynder et al. (1971), in an extensive case-control study, found no variation in blood group recorded between the prostate cancer patients and control subjects.

4.2 Ethnic Group

A number of authors have examined the prostate cancer mortality in the United States of foreign-born residents: Smith (1956) found this to be low for Japanese migrants; Haenszel (1961) found it to be reduced for whites from 12 different countries;

Haenszel and Kurihara (1968) found it reduced for Japanese; Staszewski and Haenszel (1965) found it to be low for Poles; King and Haenszel (1973) found it reduced for Chinese. Stemmerman (1970) suggested that metastatic prostatic cancer was uncommon in Japanese dying in Hawaii. Blair and Fraumeni (1978) observed that prostate cancer mortality was raised in states in the United States with a high percentage of residents from Scandinavia.

Using a variety of different approaches to examine the influence of ethnic groups on incidence or mortality from prostate cancer, Smith (1957) reported a markedly reduced mortality amongst Indians; Newill (1961) observed reduced mortality for Jews, with small differences for place of birth; Wynder et al. (1971) noted less risk of prostate cancer in immigrants from Eastern Europe; Mancuso and Stirling (1974) recorded no variation in prostate mortality for Ohio residents dying in 1959–1967 in relation to place of birth and migration within the United States; Ross et al. (1979), using cancer incidence data for Los Angeles, confirmed the very high incidence in blacks and amongst upper occupational and social class groupings.

Levine and Wilchinsky (1979) examined the stage at presentation and survival within stage of blacks versus whites. There was a significant excess of blacks with more regional and distant metastases; within stage, there was no difference for survival at 5, 10, or 15 years after treatment.

5 Association with Other Diseases

5.1 Benign Prostatic Hyperplasia

It is conceivable either that benign prostatic hypertrophy predisposes to malignant disease or that there is a factor responsible for increasing the risk of both benign and malignant disease of the prostate. The trends for mortality of these two conditions have been quite different since 1911 in England and Wales. There have been miscellaneous case reports, such as that by Guerrier and Persky (1969), who reported the association of leukaemia, hyperplasia, and carcinoma of the prostate in one patient. Armenian et al. (1974) found that there was a relative risk of 5.1 ($p < 0.001$) of finding benign prostatic hypertrophy in prostate cancer cases as against controls. In a prospective study of 345 patients with benign prostatic hypertrophy they found that the death rate from prostate cancer was 3.7 times greater following benign disease of the prostate than in the controls. However, these findings have been disputed: Franks (1974) suggested benign hypertrophy was so common it could not be directly responsible for the risk of cancer; Williams and Blackard (1974) and Rotkin (1975) felt the selection of cases and controls introduced bias in the quality of diagnosis and the use of death certificates was suspect.

Greenwald et al. (1974a) followed up over 800 patients with benign prostatic hyperplasia; there was no difference in the proportion of patients with benign hyperplasia and controls who subsequently developed prostate cancer. The British Medical Journal (1975) concluded that there was little reason to doubt the validity of the findings. Higgins (1975) suggested that latent cancers were likely to be eliminated because the benign cases were treated surgically while the controls were not (this may be a fallacious argument as resection for hyperplasia does not include the lateral lobes, in which cancer tends to occur).

5.2 Cirrhosis of the Liver

Robson (1964, 1966) examined the prevalence of prostatic cancer at autopsy of 205 patients with cirrhosis and in other autopsy subjects. A lower prevalence of prostatic cancer was found in those with severe liver disease, but no different in those patients with or without evidence of 'hyperoestrogenism'.

6 Association with Sexual Behaviour

King et al. (1963), in a lengthy review of the epidemiology of prostate cancer, concluded that sexual behaviour may be related to differences in mortality and morbidity and reflected in racial, regional, urban/rural and occupational differences.

Lancaster (1952), using mortality statistics from Australia with census data as the denominator, reported an excess of prostate cancer in married subjects who had children. A number of case-control studies have explored this issue. Wynder et al. (1971) suggested that there was no significant effect of marital status or fertility differentiating between the cases and controls. Steele et al. (1971) recorded greater extramarital activity, sexual drive, and frequency of venereal disease in the prostate cancer patients. Krain (1974) reported a significant excess of past history of venereal disease, increased coital frequency, increased number of sexual partners before marriage, and the use of contraceptive agents in the prostate cancer patients. He found no difference in the number of sexual partners after marriage. Greenwald et al. (1974b) found no difference in the marriage patterns of Harvard students subsequently dying from prostate cancer. Rotkin (1977) suggested that patients had (i) delayed sexual drive and development, (ii) repression of sexuality at the time sexual activities normally began, and (iii) a fall-off of sexuality early in adult life. No differences were found for the number of marriages or the number of sexual partners.

Schumann et al. (1977) noted a tendency amongst the prostate cancer patients for increased number of sexual partners (including prostitutes), reported prior venereal disease, and genital infections in the spouse. The age at first intercourse and first marriage was lower in the cancer patients, and the patients had higher fertility and more instances of prostate cancer among their relatives.

Greenwald et al. (1979) found no difference in the average duration of widowhood, and frequency of more than one marriage was the same for the patients with prostate cancer and controls. However, they did note an excess of breast cancer and endometrial cancer in the wives of the prostate cancer patients, though neither of these results was statistically significant.

Role of Viral Infection

One aspect of the sexual behaviour of the cases and controls is the possibility that this is associated with exposure to virus infection. Schumann et al. (1977) found slightly higher antibody titres for herpes and cytomegalic virus in prostate cancer patients than in controls. However, Ross et al. (1979) have suggested that descriptive and analytical data indicate that prostate cancer is more probably of hormonal aetiology than caused by a horizontally transmitted agent. Adequate consideration of the role of viruses is beyond this short general review; Zeigel et al. (1977) suggested that prostate cancer was one of several human cancers compatible with a viral aetiology, but much further work was required.

7 Association with Circumcision

Ravich and Ravich (1951) reported that the vast majority of their 1,400 patients with prostate obstruction were Jews; of these, only 1.8% had prostate cancer, whilst 19% of 132 non-Jews had cancer. However, because of the major biases in the referral of patients to them, it is very difficult to interpret their material. Gibson (1954) observed that 20% of 105 patients with carcinoma of the prostate had been circumcised, which he thought was a higher proportion than could be expected by chance. Of general patients referred to the three hospitals, 4.4% were Jews; of the carcinoma of the prostate patients referred for treatment, 4.2% were Jews. He suggested that the influence of circumcision was direct. Kook and Kook (1972) found only one Sefardi (Oriental) Jew compared with eight Ashkenazi (European) Jews with prostate cancer in a series of 542 males with urinary disturbances. Apt (1965) identified male groups of practising Jews in Denmark and Sweden (all of whom were circumcised); the incidence of cancer of the prostate was less than half that in the general male population. Seidman (1970) observed an appreciable difference in prostate cancer mortality between Jews and non-Jews in New York City ($p < 0.05$).
It is not clear whether some aspect of the general way of life of those orthodox members of the Jewish religion or the practice of circumcision is responsible for the observed low prostate cancer mortality in Jews.

8 Association with Other Aspects of Behaviour

8.1 Religion

Specific studies have been carried out on Seventh-day Adventists and Mormons, looking at their way of life in general and their patterns of mortality. In studies of Seventh-day Adventists, Wynder et al. (1959) observed 31 patients with prostate cancer when the figure expected was 33.75; Phillips (1975) calculated the standardised mortality ratio (SMR) for prostate cancer was 81 – or 73 when standardised for age and educational level. This still was not as marked a reduction as for other sites (many of which had SMRs of 50–70).
Enstrom (1975) observed 23 deaths from prostate cancer amongst Mormons in California in 1970–1972; three different population estimates provided expected figures which varied between 45.4 and 77.2. In a further study, Enstrom (1978) suggested that the SMR among active Mormon males in California in 1968–1975 was 79, but that among active Mormons in Utah in 1970–1975 was 107. As with the Seventh-day Adventists, prostate cancer does not show as marked a reduction as for other sites.

8.2 Social Class

Richardson (1965) obtained data from the Registrar-General in Scotland on deaths by age and social class; these showed a slightly higher death rate in the upper social classes. He also examined discharge data from hospitals; there were higher discharge rates in social classes I and II.

Seidman (1970) obtained details of the deaths in New York City and New York State for 1949–1951. Socio-economic status was defined for individuals according to their area of residence and the deaths were coded according to the religion, based on the burial ground used for the ceremony. Analysis of these data showed no clear association between socio-economic category, separated into three broad groups, and mortality from cancer of the prostate. These data were also examined within religious group, and for neither Jews nor non-Jews was there a clear relationship with socio-economic status. It is not clear whether the lack of relationship here is due to the difficulties in the method, as no more specific denominator data were available.

Ernster et al. (1977, 1978b) examined the incidence of prostate cancer and deaths in Alameda County, California in 1958–1962 and 1968–1972; area of residence was used to rank socio-economic status. They found no gradient within blacks or whites by socio-economic status. They point out that this may be due to the use of an indirect indicator of social class, under enumeration of blacks to a greater extent than white (which would result in the inflation of the black rates), and perhaps the varying influence of screening and cancer detection programmes. Ross et al. (1979) used comparable incidence data for Los Angeles County and approximately the same approach for identifying social class. These authors divided the population into five social classes and observed a significant difference between the upper and lower classes both for whites and blacks. For example, for whites they suggest that social class I had an age-adjusted incidence 23% higher than social class V.

These studies on the influence of socio-economic status on risk of prostate cancer have generally used different designs and their findings are inconsistent. It is not clear how much of this inconsistency is due to study design or whether there is a genuine small influence of social class that varies amongst different populations.

8.3 Diet

Miller (1978) reviewed hormone-associated cancers; he presented few data but suggested that variation in nutrition might be associated with hormonal differences and these could lead (i) to variation in sexual behaviour and at the same time (ii) to variation in risk of prostate cancer.

Sato (1963) suggested that those countries which have had a marked increase in prostate cancer mortality between 1952–1953 and 1958–1959 also had a marked rise in their intake of animal protein, but did not present figures to support this contention.

Takahashi (1964) found a correlation of 0.7 ($p < 0.001$) between the age-adjusted mortality for prostate cancer and coffee consumption in 20 countries. There was no similar relationship for benign prostate hyperplasia, but there was an association with prostate cancer and sugar intake.

In the 1970s a number of correlation studies examined data on food intake against a range of malignant and other diseases. Howell (1974) found an association between prostate cancer (amongst other cancers) and an index of westernisation, based on a

factor analysis of per capita food consumption. Shennan and Bishop (1974) studied 32 countries and found a correlation of 0.75 with total fat intake ($p < 0.001$). Armstrong and Doll (1975) suggested that the total fat consumption correlation was of importance, but that the previously reported relationship with coffee consumption was probably an indirect one due to the association between coffee and fat consumption. Schrauzer (1976) again found a significant correlation with fat and coffee intake (but negative correlations that were non-significant with cigarette consumption and tea drinking). Blair and Fraumeni (1978) noted that there was an elevated prostate cancer mortality in the American states where consumption of high-fat food is high.
Rotkin (1977), in his case-control study, suggested that there was elevated intake of food with appreciable lipid and cholesterol content in the prostate cancer patients compared with the controls. Wynder et al. (1971) recorded the weight and height of patients in their case-control study, but found no significant difference between the prostate cancer patients and controls. Greenwald et al. (1974b) identified no differences in indices of somatotype, gynandromorphy, androgyny, baldness, or pilosity on follow-up of a large number of Harvard students (comparing prostate cancer deaths with controls).

8.4 Smoking and Drinking

The issue of smoking and drinking has been examined in a number of the studies reported in the above section on diet. Breslow and Enstrom (1974) looked at alcohol and tobacco consumption and found that there was a non-significant relationship with prostate cancer (though beer had a consistently positive correlation). There appears to be no clear relationship between smoking or alcohol consumption and risk of prostate cancer. A number of major studies have categorised individuals by their smoking habits and then followed them up over many years to look at the patterns of mortality; for example, Doll and Peto (1976), in their 20-year follow-up of British doctors, found no excess prostate cancer in smokers.
Other evidence on the effect of alcohol is equivocal; Wynder et al. (1971) and Schoonees et al. (1972) found no relationship, whilst Pell and D'Alonzo (1973) and Schmidt and de Lint (1972) noted excess deaths from prostate cancer in follow-up studies of alcoholics. Lowenfels (1974) concluded that further study was required on larger numbers to define whether there was a hazard.

8.5 Emotion

Rotkin (1977), in his case-control study, questioned patients about various emotional trauma in their early and recent history. More of the controls had experienced broken homes during adolescence; no differences were found for indices of personality, recent stressful events, or depression prior to cancer detection.
Trunnel (1956) suggested that men who attended his hospital for prostate cancer had a constricted outlook on life, were tractable in the extreme, left most of the decisions to their wives, and had domineering wives. By intentionally upsetting patients they induced increases in serum acid phosphatase. They had also noted that when a patient became emotionally attached to another patient dying from malignant disease he would have a rise in acid phosphatase, which would increase until the death and then decrease.

9 Association with Occupation

Henry et al. (1931) examined the occupations recorded for individuals dying in England and Wales between 1921 and 1928 from cancer of the bladder and prostate. They obtained death certifications for 5,808 males dying from cancer of the prostate, and age-adjusted rates were calculated for 47 different occupations, the census data being used as a denominator. They found that several categories of open-air worker had a high SMR for prostate cancer (gardeners, farm bailiffs, agricultural labourers and shepherds, and farmers); high SMRs were also found for french-polishers, locomotive engine drivers, firemen, and cleaners. MacDonald (1956) reported a relative excess in guards and policemen, farmers, and labourers in Texas. (In contrast, there was a deficiency of skilled craftsmen in manufacturing industries, chauffeurs, firemen, and other service groups in comparison with the distribution of workers in the State.) Rotkin (1977), in his case-control study identified excess frequency of exposure to fertilisers and exhaust fumes. Detailed occupational histories were examined for some 14,000 patients admitted to Roswell Park in 1956–1965 and the relative risk for different cancers tabulated. Houten et al. (1977), using this material, found a relative risk of 6.7 for prostate cancer for blacksmiths and a risk for mechanics of 2.1 ($p < 0.05$ in both examples). Using the same basic records, Bross et al. (1978) identified a raised ratio of over 2 for dairy farmers ($p < 0.05$). Greenwald et al. (1974b), in their follow-up study of Harvard students, found that the occupations of cases and controls were similar (though occupations of Harvard graduates are likely to be very atypical).

Williams et al. (1977) presented analyses from the US Third National Cancer Survey on occupation and industry with reference to patients with different malignancies. Prostate cancer was associated with ministers, farmers, plumbers, and coal miners. Blair and Fraumeni (1978), in their examination of prostate mortality by counties in America, observed elevated rates of mortality in those with metal-using and textile industries. Ernster et al. (1979), using occupations recorded on death certificates issued in two Californian counties for patients dying of prostate cancer, found an excess reporting farming, shipfitting, compositing, and jobs entailing 'chemical exposure'.

Steele et al. (1971), in their relatively small case-control study, state that they had recorded occupation; however, in their results, they do not mention this aspect. This may be an example of the rather irritating failure to publish negative findings. (If they genuinely had screened a range of occupations and found no relationship, it would be useful if the result had actually been presented – otherwise the literature tends to be unbalanced, with publication solely of positive results or specific refutation of other work.)

9.1 Cadmium Exposure

Potts (1965) described the health of battery workers who had been exposed to cadmium oxide dust. Seventy-four men had worked for at least 10 years, eight of whom had died; three of these deaths were from prostate cancer. Though no expected figure can be calculated from these data, the proportion of prostate cancer deaths is raised. Kipling and Waterhouse (1967) surveyed 248 men who had worked for at least

1 year with cadmium oxide. The overall number of malignancies in the group was similar to that expected, but four subjects had developed prostate cancer, though the expected incidence was 0.58 ($p < 0.003$). Lemen et al. (1976) studied the mortality of men employed at a cadmium smelter in the United States; 292 men who had worked for at least 2 years between 1940 and 1969 were involved. Though there were fewer deaths in any group than expected, there was a significant excess of neoplasms (O = 27; E = 17.57; $p < 0.05$). Four deaths from prostate cancer occurred (E = 1.15); all these four occurred after a latent interval of at least 20 years from starting work.

In a case-control study Kolonel and Winkelstein (1977) observed an increased (but not significantly) risk for cadmium exposure. Ross et al. (1979) found a standardised registration ratio of 87 for 25 individuals working as photographers, painters, welders and solderers, and metal platers (i.e., occupations specifically exposing individuals to cadmium).

Kolonel (1976), in a case-control study of renal cancer, found a significant association of renal cancer with previous exposure to cadmium. Scott et al. (1976) examined clinical and biochemical aspects of coppersmiths exposed to cadmium, and compared them with non-specified assembly workers in a 'reference population'. They found a more pronounced tendency to liver damage and renal stone, and increased blood cadmium concentrations, in the coppersmiths. There was also evidence of renal impairment. The relevance of this to prostate cancer hazard was not clearly delineated.

10 Association with Environment

Richardson (1965) examined discharge data from hospitals in Scotland; there were higher discharge rates in urban than in rural areas.

Hagstrom et al. (1967) analysed the cancer mortality in the Nashville metropolitan region in 1949–1969 against indices of atmospheric pollution. There appeared to be a direct relationship between suspended particulate matter and death rates for carcinoma of the prostate; this was independent of an inverse relationship between this cancer and socio-economic class. Winkelstein and Kanto (1969) reported similar findings from New York.

11 Screening

There is little specific advice that can be given to individuals to avoid risk of prostate cancer. Mortality from this condition is still high, despite developments in treatment. This has led to a focussing of interest upon early diagnosis. In a critical review of published randomised trials of therapy for prostate cancer, Coune (1978) confirmed there was a gradient in survival from stage I to stage IV. This cannot be taken as firm evidence that early diagnosis will be of great value; the stage I/II patients may have a higher proportion of slowly growing tumours with good prognosis irrespective of delay to diagnosis. Byar (1973) suggested on the basis of results obtained in clinical trials that placebo was preferable to active treatment of localised cancer.

Gilbertsen (1971) studied nearly 6,000 men over 45 who had annual examinations including palpation of the prostate. It was suggested that the 75 patients with cancers detected by screening had better survival at 10 years (after adjustment for age of the subjects) than were recorded in the US End Results Survey (Axtell et al. 1972).

Garret and Jassie (1976) compared prostatic massage secretion smears with subsequently voided urine, and found that tests carried out with urine yielded much more accurate results. They suggested that when the urologists' findings were equivocal, such a technique might be a valuable diagnostic aid, though the role of prostatic cancer detection in symptomless subjects remains to be demonstrated. Prostatic duct carcinoma is an uncommon tumour of the prostate, but owing to the close relationship of the tumour to the urethra there is more chance of cells appearing in the voided urine. Ramzy and Larson (1977) described the cytological findings in two cases. Eposti (1971) graded the cytology from transrectal aspiration biopsy of subjects with prostate carcinoma and compared this with subsequent survival. At 5 years it was 68% for those with highly differentiated lesions, 55% for those with moderately differentiated, and 11% for those with poorly differentiated cancer. This technique is therefore satisfactory as a prognostic indicator.

Foti et al. (1977) advocated radio-immunoassay of serum acid phosphatase to screen patients for intracapsular cancer – though they were considering this for clinical rather than population screening.

A Canadian Task Force (1979) recently assessed the value of screening for many different conditions. Having considered the relatively limited evidence on prostate cancer screening based upon clinical experience and descriptive studies (rather than formal trials), they concluded that there was no evidence of efficacious treatment and prevention following digital palpation, prostatic massage and cytology, or serum acid phosphatase assay. They accepted that it might be included in a general health examination on grounds other than direct benefit from merely screening for prostate cancer.

12 Conclusions

Owen (1976), after reviewing the aetiology of prostate cancer, suggested that it was still not clear what was the effect of sexual behaviour, circumcision, zinc and cadmium, or viruses. Four years later much of the uncertainty remains and one can add to his list the role of diet and preceding benign prostatic hypertrophy. Further work on the relationship of venereal disease, other aspects of sexual behaviour, and benign prostatic hypertrophy to risk of prostate cancer is needed. There has been an expansion of various types of occupational study in recent years, and these should confirm whether or not aspects of behaviour are the important factors rather than work environment.

Studies on diet are fraught with difficulty, but research on method continues (as this topic has obvious relevance to other malignancies and many important chronic diseases). Retrospective case-control studies should be considered, but accurate

assessment of past diet is impossible; large-scale prospective studies are a daunting prospect.
The Canadian assessment seems sound: this suggests that screening for prostate cancer cannot be justified as a specific campaign, but might be introduced as part of a general health check.
The death rate from this disease remains high, and may have been increasing again in recent years – a challenge to epidemiology, early detection, and clinical care.

13 References

Akazaki K, Stemmerman GN (1973) Comparative study of the prostate among Japanese in Japan and Hawaii. J Natl Cancer Inst 50: 1137–1144

Alderson MR (1977) An introduction to epidemiology, revised reprint. Macmillan, London

Apt A (1965) Circumcision and prostate cancer. Acta Med Scand 178: 493–504

Armenian HK, Lilienfeld AM, Diamond EL, Bross IDJ (1974) Relation between benign cancer prostatic hyperplasia and cancer of the prostate. Lancet 2: 115–117

Armstrong B, Doll R (1975) Environmental factors and cancer incidence and mortality in different countries with special reference to dietary practices. Int J Cancer 15: 617–631

Axtell LM, Cutler SJ, Myers MH (eds) (1972) End results in cancer. Government Printing Office, Washington (Report no. 4, Department of Health, Education, and Welfare; Publication no. (NIH) 73-272, National Cancer Institute)

Blair A, Fraumeni JF (1978) Geographic patterns of prostate cancer in the United States. J Natl Cancer Inst 61: 1379–1384

Bourke JB, Griffin JP (1962) Blood groups in benign and malignant prostate hypertrophy. Lancet 2: 1279–1280

Breslow N, Chan CW, Dhom G, Drury RAB, Franks LM, Gellei B, Lee YS, Lundberg S, Sparke B, Sternby NH, Tullinius H (1977) Latent carcinoma of prostate and autopsy in seven areas. Int J Cancer 20: 680–688

Breslow NE, Enstrom JE (1974) Geographic correlations between cancer mortality rates and alcohol-tobacco consumption in the United States. J Natl Cancer Inst 53: 631–639

British Medical Journal (1975) Benign hyperplasia and cancer of the prostate. Br Med J 1: 2–3

Bross IDJ, Viadana E, Houten L (1978) Occupational cancer in men exposed to dust and other environmental hazards. Arch Environ Health 33: 300–307

Byar DP (1973) The Veterans Administration Cooperative Urological Research Group's studies of cancer of the prostate. Cancer 32: 1126–1130

Canadian Task Force (1979) The periodic health examination. Can Med Assoc J 121: 1193–1254

Coune A (1978) Carcinoma of the prostate. In: Staquet MJ (ed) Randomized trials in cancer: a critical review by sites. Raven Press, New York, pp 389–409

Doll R, Peto R (1976) Mortality in relation to smoking: 20 years' observation on male British doctors. Br Med J 2: 1525–1536

Edwards CN, Steinhorsson E, Nicholson D (1953) An autopsy study of latent prostate cancer. Cancer 6: 531–554

Enstrom JE (1975) Cancer mortality among Mormons. Cancer 36: 824–841

Enstrom JE (1978) Cancer and total mortality among active Mormons. Cancer 42: 1943–1951

Eposti PL (1971) Cytologic malignancy grading of prostatic carcinoma by transrectal aspiration biopsy. Scand J Urol Nephrol 5: 199–209

Ernster VL, Winkelstein W, Selvin S, Brown SM, Sacks ST, Austin DF, Mandel SA, Bertolli TA (1977) Race, socio-economic status, and prostatic cancer. Cancer Treat Rep 61: 187–191

Ernster VL, Selvin S, Winkelstein W (1978a) Cohort mortality for prostatic cancer among United States non-whites. Science 200: 1165–1166

Ernster VL, Selvin S, Sacks ST, Austin DF, Brown SM, Winkelstein JW (1978b) Prostatic cancer: mortality and incidence rates by race and social class. Am J Epidemiol 107: 311–320

Ernster VL, Selvin S, Brown SM, Sacks ST, Winkelstein W, Austin DF (1979) Occupation and prostatic cancer: a review and retrospective analysis based on death certificates in two Californian counties. Journal of Occupational Medicine 21: 175–183

Foti AG, Cooper JF, Herschman H (1977) Detection of prostatic cancer by solid-phase radioimmunoassay of serum prostatic acid phosphatase. N Engl J Med 297: 1357–1361

Franks LM (1954) Latent carcinoma of the prostate. J Pathol Bacteriol 68: 603–615

Franks LM (1956) Natural history of prostate cancer. Proceedings of the Third National Cancer Conference. Lippingcott, Philadelphia, pp 187–193

Franks LM (1974) Benign prostatic hyperplasia. Lancet 2: 293

Garret M, Jassie M (1976) Cytologic examination of post prostatic massage specimens as an aid to diagnosis of carcinoma of the prostate. Acta Cytol 20: 126–131

Gibson EC (1954) Carcinoma of the prostate in Jews and circumcised Gentiles. Br J Urol 26: 227–229

Gilbertsen VA (1971) Cancer of the prostate gland. JAMA 215: 81–84

Greenwald P, Kirmss V, Polan AK, Dick VS (1974a) Cancer of the prostate among men with benign prostatic hyperplasia. J Natl Cancer Inst 53: 335–340

Greenwald P, Damon A, Kirmss V, Polan AK (1974b) Physical and demographic features of men before developing cancer of the prostate. J Natl Cancer Inst 53: 341–346

Greenwald P, Kirmss V, Burnett WS (1979) Prostate cancer epidemiology: widowhood and cancer of spouses. J Natl Cancer Inst 62: 1131–1136

Guerrier KR, Persky L (1969) Combined leukaemia, carcinoma and hyperplasia of the prostate. Arch Surg 98: 365–366

Haenszel W (1961) Cancer mortality among the foreign born in the United States. J Natl Cancer Inst 26: 37–132

Haenszel W, Kurihara M (1968) Studies of Japanese Migrants: Mortality from cancer and other diseases among Japanese in the United States. J Natl Cancer Inst 40: 43–68

Hagstrom RM, Sprague HA, Landau E (1967) The Nashville air pollution study. VII. Mortality from cancer in relation to air pollution. Arch Environ Health 15: 237–248

Halpert B, Sheehan EE, Schmalhort WR, Scott R (1963) Carcinoma of the prostate: a survey of 5,000 autopies. Cancer 16: 737–742

Henry SA, Kennaway NM, Kennaway EL (1931) The incidence of cancer of the bladder and prostate in certain occupations. J Hyg (Camb) 30: 125–137

Henschke UK, Lasalle DL, Mason CH, Reinhold AW, Schneider RL, White JE (1973) Alarming increase of the cancer mortality in US black population (1950–67). Cancer 31: 763–768

Higgins ITT (1975) The epidemiology of cancer of the prostate. J Chronic Dis 28: 343–348

Hill GB (1975) Mortality from malignant neoplasm of the uterus since 1950. World Health Stat Rep 28: 323–338

Houten L, Bross IDJ, Viadana E, Sonnesso G (1977) Occupational cancer in men exposed to metals. Adv Exp Med Biol 91: 32–102

Howell MA (1974) Factor analysis of international cancer mortality data and per capita food consumption. Br J Cancer 29: 328–336

Jackson MA, Ahluwalia BS, Attam EB, Connolly CA, Herson J, Heshmat MY, Jackson AG, Jones GW, Kapoor SK, Kennedy J, Kovi J, Lucas AO, Nkposong EO, Olisa E, Williams AO

(1975) Characterisation of prostatic carcinoma among Blacks: a preliminary report. Cancer Chemother Rep 59: 3–15
Karube K (1961) Study of latent carcinoma of the prostate in the Japanese based on necropsy material. Tohoku J Exp Med 74: 265–285
King H, Haenszel W (1973) Cancer mortality among foreign and native-born Chinese in the United States. J Chronic Dis 26: 623–646
King H, Diamond E, Lilienfeld AM (1963) Some epidemiological aspects of cancer of he prostate. J Chronic Dis 16: 117–153
Kipling MD, Waterhouse JAH (1967) Cadmium and prostatic carcinoma. Lancet 1: 730–731
Kolonel LN (1976) Association of cadmium with renal cancer. Cancer 37: 1782–1787
Kolonel L, Winkelstein W (1977) Cadmium and prostatic carcinoma. Lancet 2: 566–567
Kook H, Kook M (1962) Carinoma of the prostate in Israel – preliminary survey. Br J Urol 34: 322–325
Krain LS (1974) Some epidemiologic variables in prostatic carcinoma in California. Prev Med 3: 154–159
Lancaster HO (1952) The mortality in Australia from cancers peculiar to the male. Med J Aust 2: 41–44
Lemen RA, Lee JS, Wagoner JK, Blejer HP (1976) Cancer mortality among cadmium production workers. Ann NY Acad Sci 271: 273–279
Levine RL, Wilchinsky M (1979) Adenocarcinoma of the prostate: a comparison of the disease in Blacks versus Whites. J Urol 121: 761–762
Lowenfels AB (1974) Alcohol and cancer. NY State J Med 74: 56–59
Lynch HT, Larsen AL, Magnuson CW, Krush AJ (1966) Prostate carcinoma and multiple primary malignancies; study of a family and 109 consecutive prostate cancer patients. Cancer 19: 1891–1897
MacDonald E (1956) Natural history of prostate cancer. Proceedings of the Third National Cancer Conference. Lippincott, Philadelphia, pp 181–185
Mancuso TF, Sterling TD (1974) Relation of place of birth and migration in cancer mortality in the US. J Chronic Dis 37: 459–474
Miller AB (1978) An overview of hormone associated cancers. Cancer Res 38: 3985–3900
Montgomery TR, Whitlock GF, Nohlgren JE, Lewis AM (1961) What becomes of the patient with latent or occult carcinoma of the prostate. J Urol 86: 655–658
Morgagni GB (1760) The seats and causes of diseases investigated by anatomy, Book 3. Johnson and Payne, London, p 460
Newill VA (1961) Distribution of the cancer mortality among ethnic sub-groups of the white population of New York City 1953–58. J Natl Cancer Inst 26: 405–417
Owen WL (1976) Cancer of the prostate – a literature review. J Chronic Dis 29: 89–114
Pell S, D'Alonzo CA (1973) A five year mortality study of alcoholics. Journal of Occupational Medicine 15: 120–125
Phillips RL (1975) Role of life-style and dietary habits in risk of cancer among Seventh-day Adventists. Cancer Res 35: 3513–3522
Potts CL (1965) Cadmium proteinuria – the health of battery workers exposed to cadmium oxide dust. Ann Occup Hyg 8: 55–61
Ramzy I, Larson V (1977) Prostatic duct carcinoma: exfoliative cytology. Acta Cytol 21: 417–420
Ravich A (1978) Point of view – misleading reports on Japanese incidence of prostatic cancer. Urology 11: 542
Ravich A, Ravich RA (1951) Prophylaxis of cancer of the prostate, penis, and cervix by circumcision. NY State J Med 51: 1519–1520
Rich AR (1935) On the frequency of the occurrence of occult carcinoma of the prostate. J Urol 33: 215–222

Richardson IM (1965) Prostatic cancer and social class. Br J Prev Soc Med 19: 140–142
Riches E (1958) Malignant disease of the urinary tract. Lancet 2: 595–598
Robson MC (1964) The incidence of benign prostatic hyperplasia and carcinoma of the prostate in cirrhosis of the liver. J Urol 92: 307–310
Robson MC (1966) Cirrhosis and prostatic neoplasms. Geriatrics 21: 150–154
Ross RK, McCurtis JW, Henderson BE, Menck HR, Mack TM, Martin SP (1979) Descriptive epidemiology of testicular and prostatic cancer in Los Angeles. Br J Cancer 39: 284–292
Rotkin ID (1975) Benign prostatic hyperplasia, prostatic cancer, and carcinogenesis. Lancet 2: 359–360
Rotkin ID (1977) Studies of the epidemiology of prostatic cancer: expanded sampling. Cancer Treat Rep 61: 173–180
Sato T (1963) Chronic disease suspected to arise through the enhanced activity of growth hormone by excessive intake of animal protein IV. The cancer and the hypertrophy of the prostate. Bulletin of the Institute of Public Health 12: 222–228
Schmidt W, De Lint J (1972) Causes of death of alcoholics. Q J Stud Alcohol 33: 171–185
Schoonees R, Polina LD, Gaete TF (1972) Prostatic carcinoma treated at categorical centre: clinical and pathological observations. NY State J Med 72: 1021–1027
Schrauzer GN (1976) Cancer mortality correlation studies. Med Hypoth 2: 39–49
Schumann LM, Mandel J, Blackard C, Bauer H, Scarlett J, McHugh R (1977) Epidemiologic study of prostatic cancer: preliminary report. Cancer Treat Rep 61: 181–186
Scott R, Mutchnik DL, Laskowski TZ, Schmalhorst WR (1969) Carcinoma of the prostate in elderly men: incidence, growth characteristics and clinical significance. J Urol 101: 602–607
Scott R, Paterson PJ, Mills EA, McKirdy A, Fell GS, Ottoway JM, Husain FER, Fitzgerald-Finch OP, Yates AJ, Lamont A, Roxburgh S (1976) Clinical and biochemical abnormalities in coppersmiths exposed to cadmium. Lancet 2: 396–398
Seidman H (1970) Cancer death rates by site and sex for religious and socio-economic groups in New York City. Environ Res 3: 234–250
Shennan DH, Bishop OS (1974) Diet and mortality from malignant disease in 32 countries. West Indian Med J 23: 44–53
Smith RL (1956) Recorded and expected mortality among the Japanese of the United States and Hawaii with special reference to cancer. J Natl. Cancer Inst 17: 460–473
Smith RL (1957) Recorded and expected mortality among the Indians of the United States with special reference to cancer. J Natl Cancer Inst 18: 385–396
Staszewski J, Haenszel W (1965) Cancer mortality among the Polish-born in the United States. J Natl Cancer Inst 35: 291–297
Steele R, Lees REM, Kraus AS, Rao C (1971) Sexual factors in the epidemiolgy of cancer of the prostate. J Chronic Dis 24: 29–37
Stemmermann GN (1970) Patterns of disease among Japanese in Hawaii. Arch Environ Health 20: 266–273
Takahashi E (1964) Coffee consumption and mortality for prostate cancer. Tohoku J Exp Med 82: 218–223
Thiessen EU (1974) Concerning a familial association between breast cancer and both prostatic and uterine malignancies. Cancer 34: 1102–1107
Trunnel JB (1956) Emotional factors in development of prostatic cancer. In: Proceedings of the Third National Cancer Conference. Lippincott, Philadelphia, pp 186–187
Tulinius H (1977) Epidemiology of prostate cancer. Recent Results Cancer Res 60: 3–13
Weiss NS (1978) Assessing the risks from menopausal estrogen use: what can we learn from trends in mortality from uterine cancer? J Chronic Dis 31: 705–708
Williams RD, Blackard CE (1974) Benign prostatic hyperplasia and cancer of the prostate. Lancet 2: 1265

Williams RR, Stegens NL, Goldsmith JR (1977) Associations of cancer site and type with occupations and industry from the Third National Cancer Survey interview. J Natl Cancer Inst 59: 1147–1185

Winkelstein W, Kantor S (1969) Prostatic cancer: relationship to suspended particulate air pollution. Am J Public Health 59: 1134–1138

Woolf CM (1960) An investigation of the familiar aspects of carcinoma of the prostate. Cancer 13: 739–743

Wynder EL, Lemon FR, Bross IJ (1959) Cancer and coronary artery disease among Seventh-day Adventists. Cancer 12: 1016–1028

Wynder EL, Maruchi K, Whitmore WF (1971) Epidemiology of cancer of the prostate. Cancer 28: 344–360

Zeigel RF, Arya SK, Horoszewicz JS, Carter WA (1977) A status report: human prostatic cancer with emphasis on potential for viral aetiology. Oncology 34: 29–44

Morphology in Health and Disease

N. J. Blacklock

Department of Urology, University of Manchester, GB – Manchester

1 Introduction

The prostate gland is a heterogeneous structure which includes glandular and fibromuscular tissue disposed around the urethra below the neck of the bladder. The glandular parenchyma lies on the posterior and lateral aspects of the urethra and is traversed on its posterior aspect by the ducts of seminal vesicles and the ampullary portions of the vasa deferentia as these pass forwards to enter the urethra in the region of the colliculus. Although the basic anatomy can be identified throughout life, there is considerable morphological change associated with the development of the mature structure in response to the stimulus of androgenic hormones and, later in life, as a result both of focal atrophy and involvement in benign hyperplastic change.
There appear to be two moieties of the functional normal adult parenchyma, and a separate origin for each of these is recognisable in embryological studies. There are possible implications of the embryological derivation in differential hormone sensitivities of each part of the gland, which may influence their differential susceptibility to disease.

2 Embryology

Glenister (1962), in a study of the development of the utricle and prostate, found that the utricular components together with the ejaculatory duct were enclosed by a condensation of mesenchyme which formed a shelf separating this part of the gland primordium from the prostatic ducts originating from the wall of the urogenital sinus below the level of the colliculus. He observed prostatic ducts to originate above the seminal colliculus, and these different levels of origin can be clearly defined in saggital sections through the prostatic urethra of the 125-mm fetus. The rudimentary prostate therefore appears to have a dual origin, so that a dual morphology in the adult may be anticipated. The site of origin of each of these entities is of significance. The primordia of the cranial entity whose ducts open into the urethra on either side of the colliculus and above it arise in the region of confluence of the urogenital sinus, the mesonephric and paramesonephric ducts. Glenister (1962) observed that the epithelium of the urogenital sinus at this site was of composite origin and derived from all three of these structures. The histological characteristics of this epithelium distinguish it from the

Recent Results in Cancer Research, Vol. 78
© Springer-Verlag Berlin · Heidelberg 1981

lining of the rest of the urogenital sinus below, which gives rise to the ducts of the lower gland entity. The glandular parenchyma developing around the ducts which arise from this composite epithelium form the cranial, central moiety of the adult gland. Since this part of the urethra is also represented in the female, this cranial part of the prostate is homologous with the female paraurethral glands or female prostate.

Andrews (1951) observed metaplasia and hyperplasia of the epithelium in the cranial, central part of the gland in the neonatal period, suggesting greater sensitivity to maternal oestrogenic stimulation. Furthermore, Huggins and Webster (1948) observed the degenerative changes in five men who had received large doses of oestrogen to be less in this part of the prostate than in the lower, more peripheral, parenchyma originating from that part of the urogenital sinus which later forms the male urethra.

These observations and the origin of the two parts of the gland suggest that there is differential steroid hormone sensitivity of the epithelium of each part.

3 Comparative Anatomy

The lower orders of mammals have a complex prostate consisting of several separate parts. The rat, which has been frequently used in prostatic research, has a prostate with ventral and paired dorsolateral and craniodorsal moieties, which cannot be directly compared with the human structure. Certain characteristics of the gland stroma or the characteristics of the secretion of each part suggest that the dorsolateral lobes are homologous with the caudal peripheral entity in the human and that the craniodorsal lobes are homologues of the more cranial central part in man. The large ventral lobe, which is convenient for experimental purposes, has no obvious homologue in either man or the non-human primate.

Study of the non-human primate shows that the baboon and various species of monkey have a bilobed prostate lying entirely behind the urethra and consisting of an upper cranial portion which is almost entirely separate from the caudal portion except at the urethral attachment of both. The upper, cranial, part has a fissured surface resembling the seminal vesicles, whereas the surface of the caudal is entirely smooth (Fig. 1). The cranial moiety surrounds both the ducts of the seminal vesicles and the common ejaculatory ducts before these enter the urethra at the colliculus. The acini of the cranial lobe are large, irregular, branching tubules with a prominent fibromuscular stroma which widely separates individual acini. The acini of the caudal lobe are smaller, consisting of simple tubules with a regular appearance overall. The appearances on conventional light microscopy and the ultrastructure of the epithelium of each moiety are distinctive (Blacklock and Bouskill 1977; Battersby et al. 1977). Van Wagenen (1936) observed that the secretion from the cranial lobe coagulated the secretion of the seminal vesicle and in this respect was similar to the secretion of the coagulating gland of the rodent, with which it may therefore be homologous. Schoonees et al. (1969) found a significantly greater concentration of zinc in the caudal lobe of the baboon prostate, and the significantly reduced concentration of zinc following castration shows that it is. The high zinc concentration of the caudal lobe resembles that in the lateral moiety of the dorsolateral prostate of the rat.

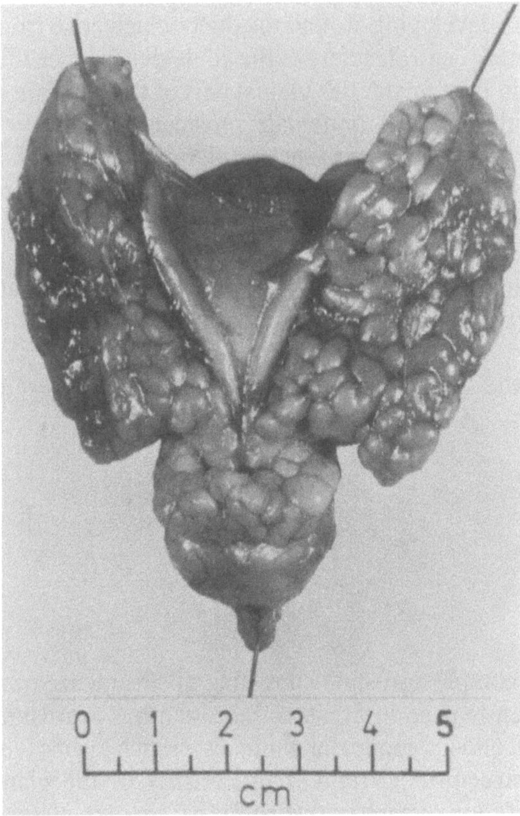

Fig. 1. Posterior aspect of bladder seminal vesicles and prostate of Rhesus monkey. The vas deferens lies medial to the seminal vesicles on each side on the back of the bladder and passes down through the fissured cranial lobe of the prostate together with the ducts of the seminal vesicles Blacklock and Bouskill 1977

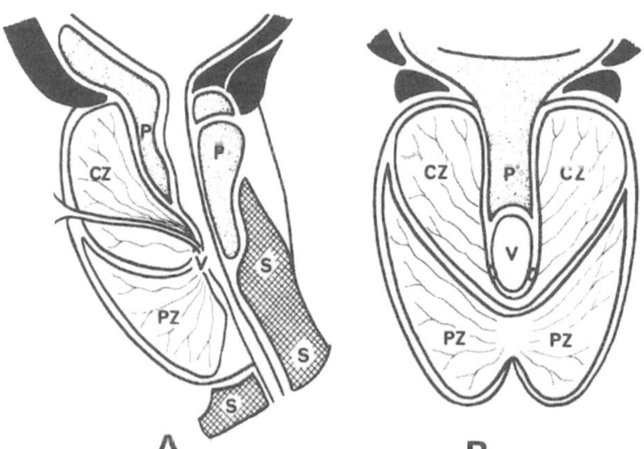

Fig. 2A, B. Diagrams of midline saggital section through the urethra **A** and coronal section behind the urethra of the human prostate **B**. *P*, pre-prostatic sphincter; *S*, striated sphincter of the urethra and external sphincter; *V*, verumontanum or colliculus; *CZ*, central zone; *PZ*, peripheral zone

4 Human Anatomy

McNeal (1968, 1972) described two subdivisions of the parenchyma of the prostate, which were comparable in many respects with those described by Hutch (1972) and broadly comparable with the original description of Lowsley (1912) if his posterior and lateral lobes were considered as one. McNeal identified a central zone cranially as being both grossly and microscopically different in appearance from a peripheral zone lying caudally and more peripheral to the central zone and partially enclosing the apex or lower end of the latter (Fig. 2). The central zone with its apex at the verumontanum or colliculus and its base above and behind the bladder neck completely surrounds the ejaculatory ducts, so that at no point do these come into contact with the peripheral zone in their course through the gland into the urethra. Tissell and Salander (1975) made a similar observation. The central zone makes up approximately a quarter of the total functional gland mass.

McNeal (1972) observed that the branching of the duct system of the central zone was more elaborate and its fibromuscular stroma more prominent and better defined. The acini are large and rectangular in cross section, with prominent intraluminal partitions. The lining epithelium is compound, with multiple layers of cells with vacuolated opaque cytoplasm. The peripheral zone has a finer stroma and a simpler form of duct branching. The acini are smaller and generally round, with a more regular epithelial lining of cells with pale, granular cytoplasm and small dark nuclei. These appearances were confirmed by Blacklock and Bouskill (1977), who also observed a tendency for the central zone to be subdivided into right and left halves.

In summary, the functional parenchyma of the human prostate external to the fibromuscular sheath surrounding the upper part of the prostatic urethra appears to have a dual morphology, which both grossly and microscopically resembles the anatomy found in the non-human primate. Glenister's observations provide the embryological derivation of each of these entities (1962).

5 Regional Pathology

The changes which lead to benign prostatic hyperplasia (BPH) occur in the submucosal glands beneath the neck of the bladder (subcervical position) and in the submucosal glands, the fibromuscular stroma of the peri-urethral sphincter of the upper part of the prostatic urethra (preprostatic sphincter, McNeal 1972) and a 'transitional zone' just external to the lower, anterolateral extremity of this sphincter (McNeal 1978) (Figs. 3 and 4). The development of hyperplasia in these positions gives rise to the typical adenomatous protrusions which are found in the fully developed case of BPH. Bilateral, anterolateral hyperplasia is most common, but there is usually also some element of subcervical hyperplasia (Figs. 5 and 6). The hyperplasia in this latter position can assume large proportions with extension into the cavity of the bladder and displacement of the lower ends of the ureters (Fig. 7). The integrity of the preprostatic sphincter may be destroyed in greater or lesser degree but remains, at least peripheral to the adenoma, as part of its capsule, which separates it from the central and peripheral zone of the functional parenchyma externally.

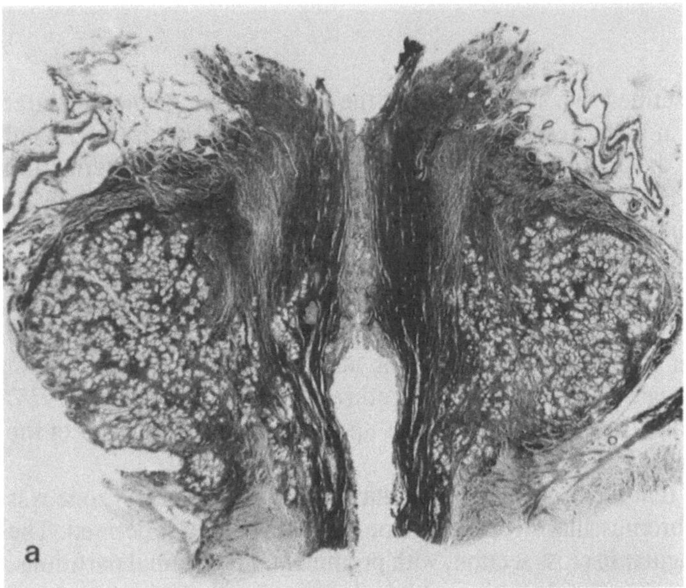

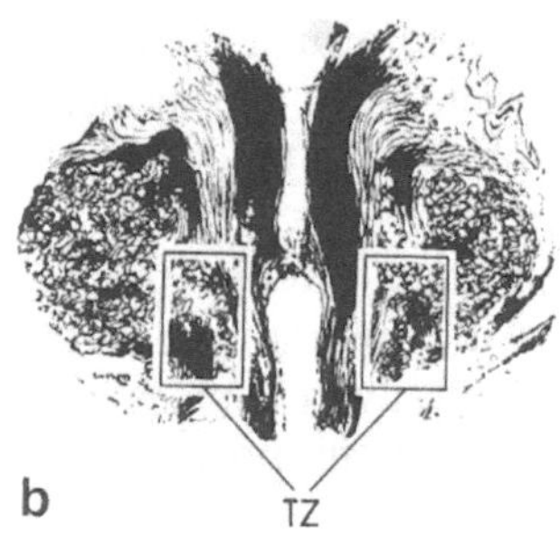

Fig. 3a, b. Coronal section through the urethra, showing the location of the structures involved in the origins of BPH: submucosal glands, preprostatic sphincter, and transitional zone with the functional parenchyma lying external to these structures. *TZ*, transitional zone

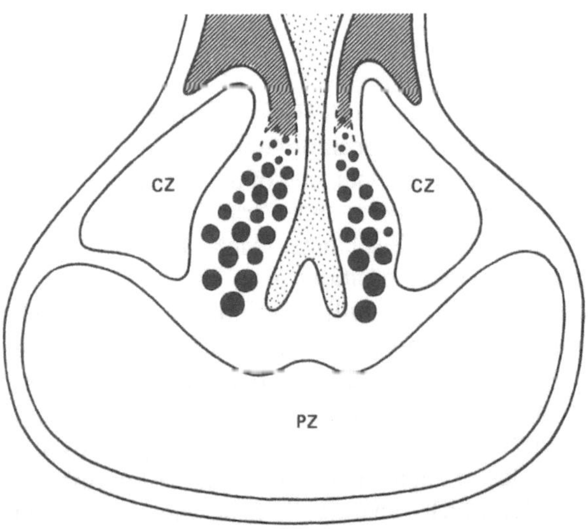

Fig. 4. Diagram of coronal section through the prostate, showing the locations of origin of BPH in the submucosal glands, preprostatic sphincter and 'transitional zone' (McNeal 1978) and its relationship to both the prostatic urethra above the verumontanum and the tissues of the central and peripheral zones

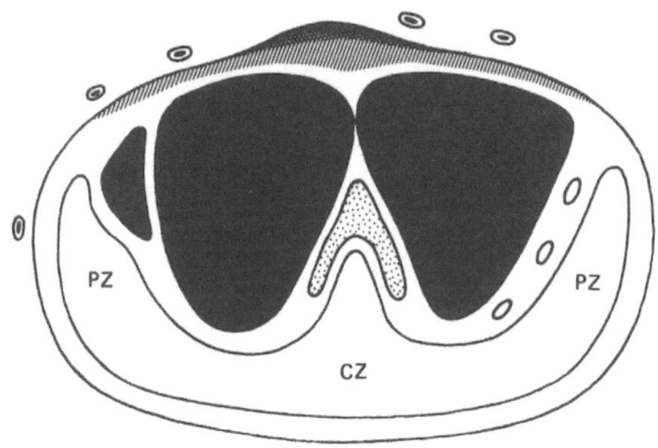

Fig. 5. Diagram of cross section of the prostate at verumontanum, showing characteristic distribution of fully developed BPH and its relationship to the urethra and the functional BPH and its relationship to the urethra and the functional prostate, which is pushed in a posterior direction

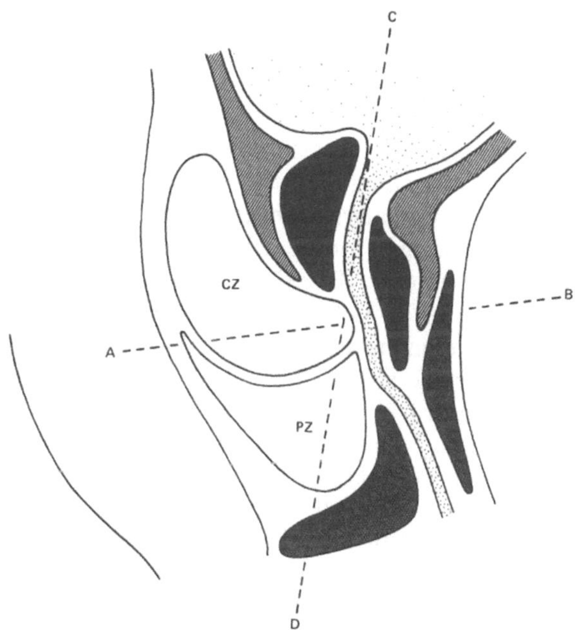

Fig. 6. Diagram of midline saggital section through the bladder neck, prostate, and membranous urethra showing relationship of BPH (in black) to the urethra, neck of the bladder, and functional prostate represented by central and peripheral zones. *AB*, plane of cross section of prostate at the level of the verumontanum; *CD*, plane of coronal section in the line of the urethra above but passing through the peripheral zone of the prostate below

Prostatitis, atrophy, and carcinoma occur commonly in the peripheral zone of the functional parenchyma (McNeal 1968). McNeal observed that prostatitis was more frequent in the peripheral than in the central zone, even allowing for the greater size of the former. In only two of forty instances did he find inflammation confined to the central zone.

Atrophic change of the columnar acinar epithelium with replacement by lower cuboidal or flattened cells was observed more often in the peripheral than in the central zone (McNeal 1968). These changes are accompanied by diminution of the complement of secretory granules and vacuolation. Similar appearances have been observed in the epithelium of castrated men and in those who have received treatment with oestrogens. The observation by Chandler et al. (1975) that zinc is present within these secretory granules is significant when considered with Schoonees (1969)

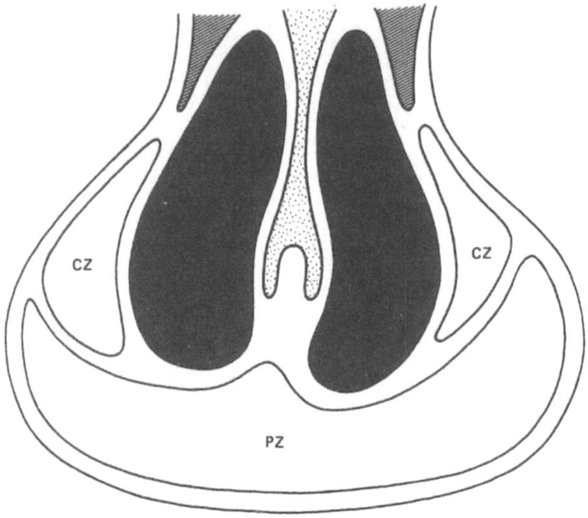

Fig. 7. Diagram of coronal section, showing the relationship of fully developed BPH to the urethra, the verumonantum, the neck of the bladder, and the functional prostate represented by the central and peripheral zones

observations that the zinc content of the caudal lobe of the baboon diminishes following castration.

The relatively greater dependence of the peripheral zone epithelium on testosterone is thought to account for the delay observed in the development of the peripheral zone acini until puberty (Blacklock 1976), and this is supported by the observation by Ghanadian et al. (1977) that there is a significantly greater number of androgen receptor sites in the monkey caudal lobe, which is the morphological homologue of the human peripheral zone.

Carcinoma of the prostate arises particularly in the peripheral zone (McNeal 1968), although it may be multifocal within this zone and spread to involve other parts of the prostate, including areas of hyperplasia, and ultimately the urethra. Carcinoma in situ has also been observed within hyperplastic nodules of the prostate, and this entity appears to differ biologically from the neoplasia arising in the peripheral zone. There are as yet no observations of how frequently the parenchyma of the central zones gives origin to cancer. The central zone therefore appears less implicated in prostatitis and less susceptible to atrophy, whilst its role in neoplasia is unknown.

The peripheral location of prostatic cancer accounts for some of the clinical features of the disease. In this position, early spread through the capsule into surrounding tissues may occur and the urethra is not immediately implicated, so that obstructive symptoms are unusual in the earlier stages of the disease.

6 Clinical and Research Implications

The genesis of BPH in the positions already described emphasises the intimate relationship it has with the prostatic urethra and provides the reason for the frequency of disturbed micturition in this disease.

Benign prostatic hyperplasia may be dealt with either by open (transvesical or retropubic) prostatectomy or by perurethral resection. With either technique the hyperplastic tissue is removed and only rarely is the functional parenchyma lying peripherally and posteriorly encroached upon. This, however, is often reduced to a thin rim of tissue. It is therefore unlikely that focal carcinoma within the prostate will be detected either in the enucleated or in the resected specimen of hyperplastic tissue, except in the instance of carcinoma in situ within the hyperplasia or where neoplasia in the peripheral zone has infiltrated into the nodule. Similarly, where neoplasia is suspected transurethral resection may fail to provide neoplastic tissue for histological confirmation. Knowledge of the anatomy shows the necessity of either perineal or transrectal biopsy of the peripheral zone of the gland to provide the best chance of encountering neoplasia.

These features of both the normal and the pathological morphology of the gland are relevant in the context of research when tissue culture and cell kinetic techniques are contemplated. Studies using these techniques have frequently used hyperplastic tissue, the biological characteristics of whose epithelium and stroma probably differ considerably from those of the tissue of the functional parenchyma, either in the peripheral or in the central zone. From all the evidence – embryological, developmental, and functional – it is likely that the biological characteristics of the epithelium of each of these zones are also distinctive.

7 References

Andrews GS (1951) The histology of the human foetal and pre-pubertal prostates. J Anat 85: 44–54

Battersby S, Chandler JA, Harper ME, Blacklock NJ (1977) The ultrastructure of Rhesus monkey prostate. Urol Res 5: 175–183

Blacklock NJ (1976) Surgical anatomy of the prostate. In: Innes Williams D, Chisholm GD (eds) Scientific foundations of urology. Heinemann, London, pp 313–315

Blacklock NJ, Bouskill K (1977) The zonal anatomy of the prostate in man and in the Rhesus monkey. Urol Res 5: 163–167

Chandler JA, Harper ME, Blundell GK, Morton MS (1975) Examination of the subcellular distribution of zinc in rat prostate after castration using the electron microscope microanalyser (EMMA). J Endocrinol 65: 34–35

Ghanadian R, Smith CB, Chisholm GD, Blacklock NJ (1977) Differential androgen uptake by the lobes of the Rhesus monkey prostate. Br J Urol 49: 701–704

Glenister TW (1962) The development of the utricle and of the so called "middle" or "median" lobe of the human prostate. J Anat 96: 443–455

Huggins C, Webster WO (1948) Duality of the human prostate in response to oestrogens J Urol 59: 258–266

Hutch JA (1972) Anatomy and physiology of the bladder, trigone and urethra. Butterworths, London, p 236

Lowsley OS (1912) The development of the human prostate gland with reference to the development of other structures in the neck of the urinary bladder. Am J Anat 13: 299–349

McNeal JE (1968) Regional morphology and pathology of the prostate. Am J Clin Pathol 49: 347–357

McNeal JE (1972) The prostate and prostatic urethra: a morphologic synthesis. J Urol 107: 1008–1016

McNeal JE (1978) Origin and evolution of benign prostate enlargement. Invest Urol 15: 340–345

Schoonees R, de Klerk JN, Murphy GP (1969) Correlation of prostatic blood flow with ^{65}Zinc activity in intact, castrated and testosterone-treated baboons. Invest Urol 6: 476–484

Tissell LE, Salander H (1975) The lobes of the human prostate. Scand J Urol Nephrol 9: 185–191

Van Wagenen G (1936) The coagulating function of the cranial lobe of the prostate gland in the monkey. Anat Rec 66: 411–414

Growth Kinetics

M. R. Alison and N. A. Wright

Department of Histopathology, Royal Postgraduate Medical School, Hammersmith Hospital, Ducane Road, GB – London W12 OHS

1 Introduction

The growth rate of a tumour can only be measured if the size can be accurately recorded on two or more occasions. The impracticability of performing such in vivo measurements, of required precision, upon prostate glands has therefore precluded any direct estimates of how fast such tumours grow. A large proportion of cell kinetic studies of the prostate gland have been carried out upon excised tumour specimens or in organ culture. Valuable cell kinetic techniques, such as the percentage of labelled mitoses method for measuring the intermitotic time of proliferating cells, are readily performed in animals (Alison and Wright 1979a), but the necessary repeated sampling over a prolonged interval is not feasible in human subjects, particularly in an ageing population. The lack of any direct estimates of growth rate means that we can only speculate upon the respective roles of cell production and cell loss in determining overall tumour growth rates.

2 Prostate Cancer

2.1 Mitotic Rate and Thymidine Labelling

The most direct evidence of population growth is the observation of dividing cells, and their relative number expressed as a proportion of the total number of cells is the mitotic index. The mitotic index is, however, a rather crude cell kinetic parameter: high values could result from a high cell production rate or from an extended duration of mitosis itself, or from a combination of the two. However, we sought a correlation between the mitotic index and the histopathological grade of the prostatic tumour cells counted. It must be strongly emphasised that this rigid classification applies only to those cells actually counted; invariably there have been glandular elements of a different type in separate areas of the same gland, but these are not counted. Furthermore, the heterogeneity of tumour type within most glands has often been considered a bar to grading such tumours (Byar and Mostofi 1972). The mitotic index data are shown in Fig. 1, and suggest that some of the more poorly differentiated tumour types have higher cell production rates than the majority of moderately to well-differentiated tumours. A single example of papillary carcinoma, classified as

Recent Results in Cancer Research, Vol. 78
© Springer-Verlag Berlin · Heidelberg 1981

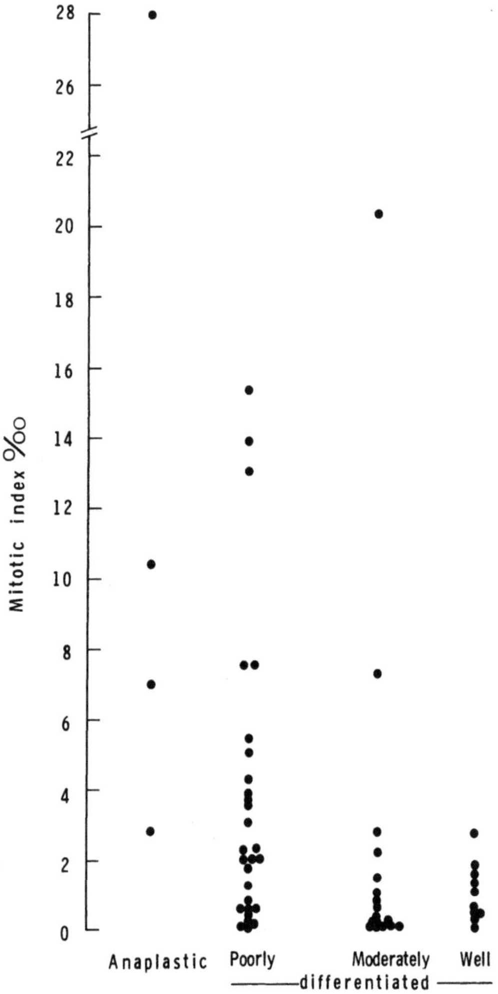

Fig. 1. The mitotic index in human prostatic adenocarcinomas of differing histopathological type. Each value was derived by counting 6,000 cells from similar areas within each tumour

moderately differentiated, had a mitotic index of 2%. In the poorly differentiated tumours, the highest mitotic indices were observed when the cells were predominantly in sheets, whilst the lowest values were commonly found when cells occurred in streams infiltrating the stroma.

The interpretation of results from this type of study depends not only upon the accurate assessment of the duration of mitosis, but also on the age structure of the tumour cell population. If the absolute cell production rate is constant and therefore the population growth curve is linear, in the absence of cell loss the time needed to double the population is also equal to the turnover time (T_t) in the population, which is the time required to replace all the cells:

$$T_t = \frac{t_M}{MI}$$

where t_m is the duration of mitosis and MI is the mitotic index. Alternatively, the cell production rate may remain in constant relation to the population size and therefore make growth exponential; in such a case the potential doubling time (T_{pot}) is a fraction

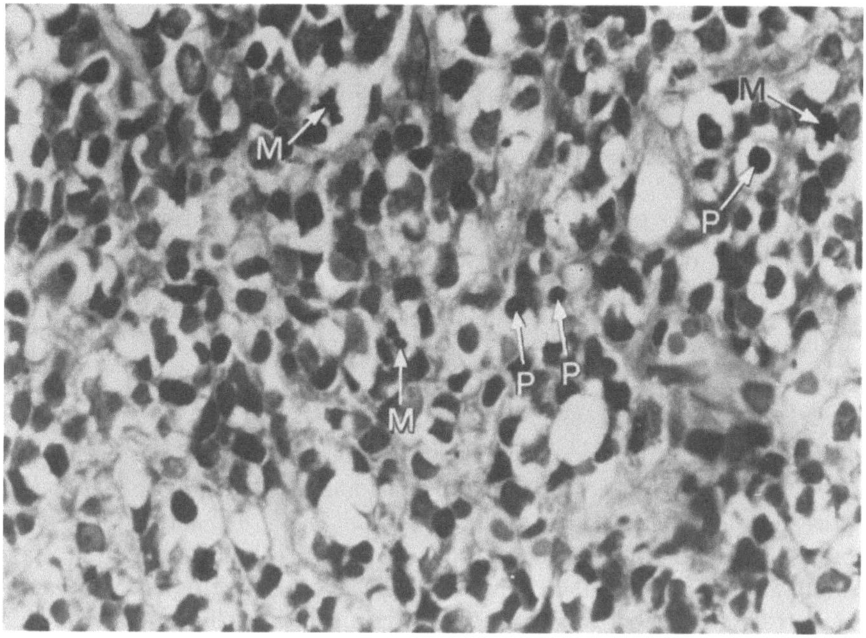

Fig. 2. Area of rather poorly differentiated prostatic adenocarcinoma illustrating the frequent appearance of mitotic figures (*M*) and pyknotic nuclei (*P*). H and E, 720×

(0.693) of the turnover time, since there will be a preponderance of young cells which remain to enlarge the pool of proliferating cells (see Aherne et al. 1977). In this instance, the choice between linear and exponential growth is probably less significant than the duration of mitosis in calculation of the population doubling time. The duration of mitosis is difficult to estimate, but is commonly between 1 and 2 h in mammalian cells (Cleaver 1967). If we assume exponential growth and $t_m = 2$ h, the population doubling time would be just over 2 days for a population with a mitotic index of 2.8% from which no cell loss was occurring.

A population doubling time of 2 days is never found because cell production is only one facet of growth, and it is its competition with cell loss which determines overall tumour growth rates. Cell loss occurs by various routes; hypoxia and karyotypic abnormalities (see Sect. 2) may be particularly important in this respect. The apparently higher cell production rates in the more poorly differentiated tumours may be counteracted by higher cell loss rates; evidence of cellular death was consistently more apparent in this group of tumours (Fig. 2). The potential doubling time is most commonly estimated by measurement of the thymidine labelling index (I_s) and the duration of the period of DNA synthesis (t_s) according to the relationship

$$T_{\mathrm{pot}} = \lambda \frac{t_s}{I_s}$$

where λ is a parameter of the age distribution of an exponential population (Steel 1977). Its minimum value is 0.693 and it increases as the S phase moves nearer to the beginning of the cell cycle. The labelling index is normally a larger fraction than the mitotic index because $t_s > t_m$, usually by a factor of 5–10. It follows that the labelling

Table 1. Thymidine labelling data from human prostate gland

Type	I_s (%)	t_s (h)[a]	Source
Poorly differentiated adenocarcinoma	1.1–3.8	8	Helpap et al. (1974)
Well-differentiated adenocarcinoma	0.4–1.9	8	Helpap et al. (1974)
Hyperplastic epithelium	0.1–0.6	10–15	Stiens et al. (1975)
Epithelium adjacent to inflammation (prostatitis)	1.2–2.1	10–15	Stiens et al. (1975)
Squamous metaplasia	4.3	11.8	Helpap and Stiens (1975)

[a] Estimated by double thymidine labelling (Wimber 1963)

index will have a smaller relative error. Thymidine labelling has been performed in vitro on excised prostatic tumour specimens, and the data are summarized in Table 1. Poorly differentiated tumours in which $I_s = 3.8\%$, $t_s = 8$ h, and $\lambda = 0.75$ would have a potential doubling time of almost 7 days. Steel (1977) has pointed that the expected doubling times of all the tumours that have been studied are very short in comparison with their actual doubling times, and concluded that cell loss was an important determinant of any tumour growth rate.

A correlation between histopathological type or stage and potential doubling time has been sought in other tumour types. Adopting metaphase arrest techniques, Fulker et al. (1971) reported that the loss of differentiation in carcinomas of the urinary bladder was associated with shorter potential doubling times, whilst Camplejohn et al. (1973) failed to find a correlation between the potential doubling time and the clinical (Dukes) stage of human rectal carcinomas.

2.2 DNA Analysis of Cells in Tumours

The measurement of nuclear DNA content can give the fraction of cells in the S, G_2, and M phases of the cell cycle. In populations of tumour cells, varying degrees of aneuploidy obscure the derivation of such kinetic information. Two techniques have been commonly applied to fine-needle aspiration biopsy specimens from the prostate gland. These are firstly the relatively laborious microdensitometric analysis of Feulgen-stained preparations, and secondly the more recent application of high-speed flow systems for automated single-cell analysis of the DNA content in large populations of cells. The two techniques have largely led to the same conclusions; hyperplastic glands and well-differentiated adenocarcinomas are predominantly composed of homogeneous populations of diploid cells (Zetterberg and Esposti 1976; Bichel et al. 1977), indicating little proliferative activity and few cytological abnormalities. The more poorly differentiated tumours have an increased frequency of aneuploidy (Frederiksen et al. 1978). Moderately differentiated tumours fall into two groups: those which consist almost totally of diploid cells and those which have considerable numbers of tetraploid and octaploid cells (Zetterberg and Esposti 1976; Bichel et al. 1977). Poorly differentiated tumours commonly have large numbers of cells in the tetraploid and octaploid regions (Fig. 3). The scarcity of mitotic figures in

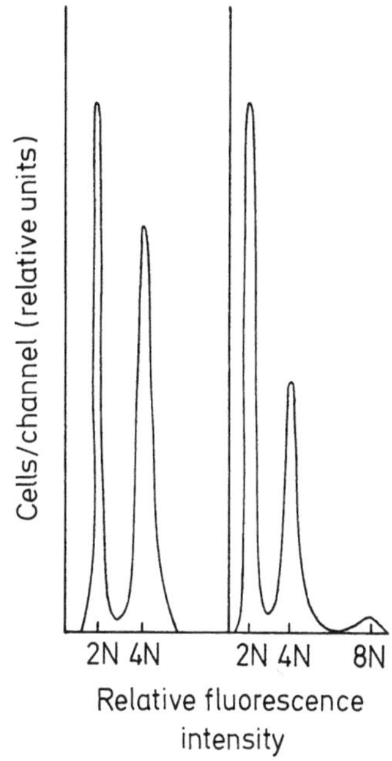

Fig. 3. Flow microfluorometric analysis of cellular DNA content in two cases of poorly differentiated prostatic cancer. Redrawn from Bichel et al. (1977)

all these studies was considered to indicate that cells with ploidy values > 2 N were cytologically abnormal.

It is clear that in many malignant tumours an abnormal DNA content per nucleus represents an abnormal chromosome complement (Spriggs 1976). Aneuploidy appears to be increasingly associated with a loss of differentiation in prostatic tumours, so that cell death due to defective mitotic mechanisms may be a significant route of cell loss. As mentioned above, higher cell production rates may be counteracted by high cell loss rates in these poorly differentiated tumours. The situation appears to be analogous to that of transitional cell carcinoma of the urinary bladder, wgere only the poorly differentiated neoplasms have abnormally high chromosome numbers (Spooner and Cooper 1972) and these same tumours have the highest cell production rates (Fulker et al. 1971). From the clinical viewpoint the main purpose of flow-cytometric analyses of DNA is to diagnose prostatic cancer, rather than to measure the proportion of cells in the S, G_2, and M phases of the cell cycle. The diagnostic significance of nuclear DNA measurements has recently been questioned because of the presence of proliferating inflammatory cell populations in many benign lesions (Sprenger and Witte 1979). On the other hand, a method has recently been described to facilitate the removal of the inflammatory mononuclear cells from the analysis of epithelial cells (Collste et al. 1979).

2.3 Studies in Culture

The term 'stem cell' refers to those cells which have the capacity to produce a large family of descendants within their natural environment. It is a functional concept, for the investigation of stem cells must necessarily involve techniques based upon the capacity of isolated cells, in an artificial environment, to produce a large family of

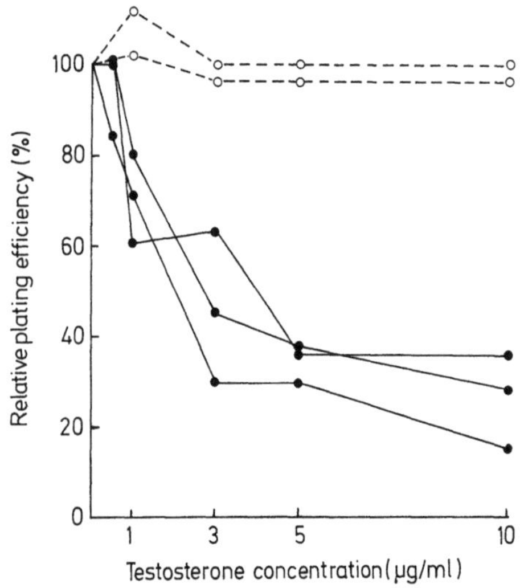

Fig. 4. Changes in the cloning ability of cells derived from benign prostatic hyperplastic explants (●) and prostatic cancer explants (○) when the soft agar culture medium was supplemented with increasing concentrations of testosterone. Redrawn from Brehmer et al. (1972)

descendants – a *clone.* A clonogenic cell assay technique based on soft agar in vitro culture has been employed for monolayer outgrowths from benign and malignant prostatic explants (Brehmer et al. 1972). Cells derived from hyperplastic tissue had plating efficiencies ranging from 6%–15%, whilst cells from adenocarcinoma of the prostate had efficiencies of 22%–27%. These very high plating efficiences contrast with the relatively low values obtained (0.001%–1%) when a variety of human cancers have been cloned directly in soft agar (Hamburger and Salmon 1977; Hamburger et al. 1978). Figure 4 illustrates the changes in plating efficiency when the soft agar was supplemented with testosterone. We can speculate that cells from benign tissue may succumb to a differentiating influence of testosterone, and differentiation by a negative feedback mechanism inhibits proliferation and therefore clone development. If this concept is correct, then cancer cells appear to be immune to such hormonal influences. A differential effect in cell culture has also been described in response to interferon (Chawda et al. 1979). Interferon inhibited the uptake of thymidine into fibroblast-like cells derived from benign hyperplastic explants, but caused no inhibition in cells derived from malignant tissue.

The response of cultured prostatic cancer tissue to hormonal influences may be dependent upon the state of differentiation. McMahon et al. (1972) reported that whilst a moderately differentiated tumour was directed towards further differentiation by testosterone, an anaplastic tumour, though showing some tendency to form acini, responded to testosterone principally by a fourfold increase in the number of mitoses observed per high-power field.

2.4 Experimental Prostatic Tumours

Most tumours in experimental animals grow appreciably faster than those in man; exponential prostatic tumours appear to be no exception. The slow growth rate of many human tumours indicates the presence of important growth restraints; these would appear to be lacking in most experimental prostatic tumours, although a volume-doubling time of 20 days is considered a slow growth rate by some investigators. Table 2 illustrates some of the data available from the most widely

Table 2. Adenocarcinomas of the prostate gland in rats

Strain	Histology[a]	Androgen dependence	Doubling time (days)	Source
Aged germ-free Wistar	Mixed	+	–	Pollard (1973)
Aged AxC	Mixed	+	10–22 months to attain 0.5–5 cm^3	Shain et al. (1979)
Noble	MD	+	$\simeq$ 6	Drago et al. (1979a)
Noble	PD	–	$\simeq$ 12	Drago et al. (1979a)
Copenhagen	WD	+	$\simeq$ 20	Isaacs et al. (1978)
Copenhagen	WD	–	$\simeq$ 20	Isaacs et al. (1978)
Copenhagen	Anaplastic	–	$\simeq$ 2	Weissman et al. (1977)

[a] WD, well-differentiated; MD, moderately differentiated; PD, poorly differentiated

studied rat prostate adenocarcinomas; their popularity stems from the fact that they mimic many of the features seen in human disease. Spontaneous adenocarcinomas arising in 70% of AxC strain rats over 24 months of age, coupled with a slow growth rate, appear to warrant most attention. Despite the relatively rapid growth rates of many of these tumours, it is perhaps surprising that no data have been forthcoming on the respective roles of cell production and cell loss in determining overall tumour growth rates.

Rao et al. (1978) have described an in vitro clonogenic cell assay for the rapidly growing anaplastic tumour in Copenhagen rats. Cells were cultured directly from the tumour and had a plating efficiency of 4%. Tumour xenographs have also been performed: prostatic cancer tissue from both rats (Drago et al. 1979b) and man (Hindsley et al. 1978) have been propagated in immunologically deprived mice, but no growth kinetic data were presented.

3 Benign Prostatic Hyperplasia

3.1 Mitotic Rate and Thymidine Labelling

In benign prostatic hyperplasia, the only proliferatively active cells are thought to reside in the basal cell region. Basal or reserve cells, which are easily recognizable in the prostate gland of both man (Dermer 1978) and dog (Timms et al. 1976), lie between the luminal columnar epithelium and the basement membrane of glandular acini. During a period of 24 h in organ culture, Dermer (1978) observed that only the basal cells incorporated tritiated thymidine, although only 0.1% cells became labelled. Slightly higher labelling indices have been found when tissue has been incubated with thymidine immediately after excision (Table 1). The close proximity of inflammation, and of oestrogen-induced squamous metaplasia, increased thymidine labelling, but in both instances labelling was confined to the basal cell region. Mitotic figures occur very infrequently in hyperplastic epithelium. To increase the mitotic index in hyperplastic prostates, Liavag (1968) injected the mitotic arresting agent Colcemid into his patients 4.5 h before excision. Despite this procedure, on average only 163 metaphases were found in the hyperplastic and atrophic glands from 10 g tissue. Farnsworth and Montes (1979) have suggested that the epithelial cell index in benign prostates is about 30%; this would mean that 10 g tissue has 3×10^9 epithelial cells. If this is correct, and assuming Colcemid caused a linear increase in metaphases with time, the turnover time for the epithelium in benign prostatic hyperplasia could be many years.

3.2 Studies in Tissue Culture

A number of organ culture studies have been concerned with evaluating the effects of hormones upon hyperplastic tissue. Morphological integrity appears to be retained in vitro in the absence of all hormones (Lasnitzki et al. 1975) and in the presence of insulin-supplemented media only (McMahon and Thomas 1973; McRae et al. 1973). Although growth did occur in the absence of androgens, the tissues may remain sensitive to hormonal manipulation; Lasnitzki et al. (1975) observed that both testosterone and 5α-dihydrotestosterone enhanced the uptake of ^{3}H-uridine, whilst McRae et al. 1973 noted an increase in DNA concentration in some testosterone-supplemented cultures.

A further common observation is that proliferative rates increase in short-term organ culture. The uptake of labelled nucleotides into DNA reaches peak values after 3–4 days of organ culture (McMahon and Thomas 1973; Shipman et al. 1975). Using the metaphase-arresting agent Vincristine, Shipman et al. (1975) observed that a 4-h blockade accumulated approximately twice as many metaphases on day 4 of culture as it did on day 2. Although linearity of accumulation was not proven, or claimed, the data suggest that the doubling time for the epithelium decreased from 30 days to 15 days between day 2 and day 4 of culture. A diversity of tissues show a mitotic response after explantation, so it seems improbable that the response seen in the human prostate is directly concerned with hormonal deprivation. It is possible that the response represents a more fundamental alteration in the control of cell division; clearly in vivo the prostate is subject to important growth-restraining influences.

4 Androgens and the Cell Cycle

4.1 The Growth Fraction

The use of the term cell cycle time has led to a certain amount of confusion in the prostate literature. Tuohimaa and Niemi (1968) concluded from a knowledge of the labelling index (1.3%) and the duration of DNA synthesis (12 h) that the cell cycle time in the seminal vesicle of castrated mice was 900 h. Implicit in the cell cycle concept is the idea of continuous progression through a chain of events leading to division; the experimental data from slowly proliferating populations cannot be reconciled to such a concept, and indicate that this progress can be arrested at some

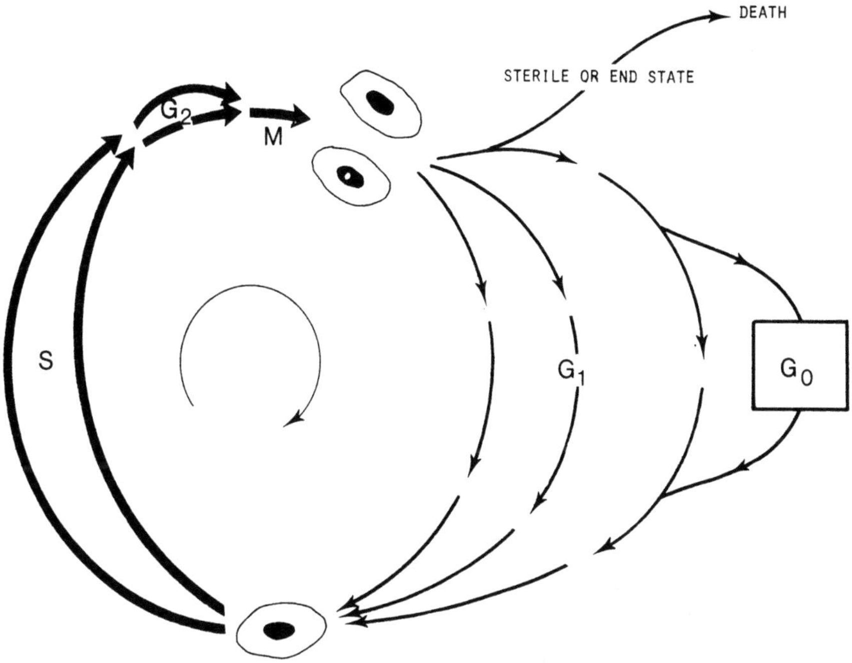

Fig. 5. Possible variations of residence time in the various phases encompassed within the life history of a cell

stage. The parameter calculated by Tuohimaa and Niemi (1968) was not the cell cycle time, but the turnover time (see Sect. 2.1). The turnover and potential doubling time of cell populations can only be equated with the cell cycle time when the whole population is in the actual division cycle (Fig. 5), i.e., when the *growth fraction* is unity. The term 'cell cycle timc', referring to the interval between successive mitoses, can also be objected to. A preferred alternative is 'intermitotic time', for the term 'cycle' implies regularity, and many populations have cells proceeding through the division sequence at markedly different rates (Alison and Wright 1979a).

Figure 5 illlustrates possible variations of residence time in the various phases encompassed in the division sequence. In studying populations with a low proliferative rate it may be difficult to distinguish between cells slowly progressing through the division sequence (particularly G_1) and those cells actually 'arrested' or 'resting' in a separate phase, designated G_0. This problem of definition should at least be appreciated when we describe a slowly proliferating population as possibly having a low growth fraction, i.e., a low proportion of cells actively proceeding towards division. Further discussion (see Sect. 4.2) presents evidence that most cells in prostatic tissues are in a state of proliferative rest (G_0), and that increased cell production is achieved by actively promoting G_0 cells into the division sequence.

4.2 Stimulated DNA Synthesis

The proliferative rate of rodent prostatic tissues can be dramatically increased if, after a period of castration-induced androgen deprivation sufficient to cause abnormal cell loss, testosterone is administered. One of the characteristics of this process is a

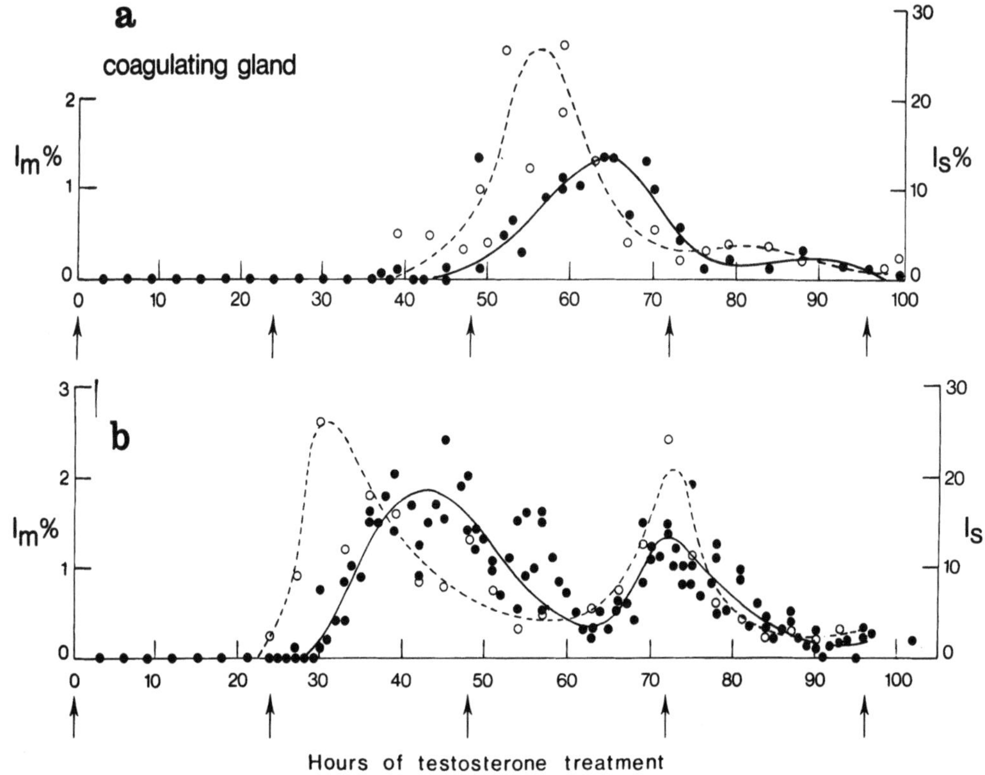

Fig. 6a, b. Labelling index (○) and mitotic index (●) in the coagulating gland of the castrated male Balb/c mouse during daily treatment with 250 μg testosterone propionate (*arrows*). Treatment commencing 3 days (**a**) and 14 days (**b**) after castration. Alison and Wright (1979a)

time-lag of 15–40 h before the stimulated cells enter DNA synthesis. This time-lag has become known as the *prereplicative phase,* and is the interval required to allow the build-up of the necessary biochemical machinery for the division sequence. Much attention has been given to this phase in an attempt to understand the fundamentals of the mechanism of action of androgens. Briefly, testosterone is first metabolised to a variety of metabolites, principally 5α-dihydrotestosterone, within the target cells (Alison and Wright 1979b). Dihydrotestosterone and possibly testosterone are then transferred to the chromatin by a receptor-mediated mechanism (see review by King and Mainwaring 1974). The association of hormone-receptor complexes and chromatin results in the phosphorylation of chromosomal non-histone proteins, and this may lead to specific gene derepression or gene activation (Ahmed and Wilson 1978). Rapid increases in RNA synthesis are ultimately followed by synthesis of the proteins necessary for DNA synthesis and mitosis (Mainwaring 1977).

The testosterone-induced proliferative response in the coagulating gland of the castrated mouse has been monitored by serial measurements of the thymidine labelling index and mitotic index. The response ensuing in mice castrated just 3 days prior to testosterone treatment (Fig. 6a), has been compared with that in mice castrated 14 days prior to testosterone treatment (Fig. 6b). The differences in magnitude of response are a reflection of the cell production required to restore the precastration cellularity of the glands (Alison and Wright 1979a). The most significant finding was that the prereplicative period, the interval between testosterone administration and the initiation of DNA synthesis, was not immutable and became substantially shorter in the longer-term castrated mice. A state of physiological quiescence ensues with time after castration, including falls in RNA and protein synthesis, 5α-reductase levels, and androgen receptor concentrations, yet such changes are paralleled by a more rapid 'switch-on' of DNA synthesis once the stimulus is applied. Baserga (1976) has suggested that cells may pass into different 'depths' of G_0, because it was observed that the prereplicative period of cultured fibroblasts, stimulated by a nutritional change, became longer as the interval between confluence and stimulation was delayed. The coagulating gland appears to behave in an opposite manner, with cells apparently moving at a 'shallower level within G_0' with the longer period of physiological quiescence resulting from androgen deprivation.

Cell proliferation can clearly be stimulated by testosterone, yet the level at which proliferative rate is ultimately maintained must be largely independent of hormonal influences. Once the accessory sex glands of castrated rodents reach precastration cellularity under the influence of androgens, cell proliferation is 'switched off', despite the continued administration of very large doses of androgen. Muntzing et al. (1979) suggested there was no evidence of a local growth inhibitor in the ventral prostate of intact rats, because implantation of atrophied prostate subsequently caused a substantial increase in the DNA content of the gland. Alison et al. (1979) observed that the extent of cell production in paired sex glands was controlled by each gland individually, consequently independently of its contralateral partner, and not by the total mass of homologous tissue in the paired glands.

The pattern of re-entry into the division sequence indicates that the slow proliferative rate of glands in intact or castrated mice was due to cells being arrested or resting at some point in the G_1 phase, or in a G_0 phase. The temporal relationships of the resumption in DNA synthesis and that of mitosis indicate that *all* cells must begin some distance from the G_1-S boundary, and then proceed through the S and G_2 phases before dividing.

4.3 Some Properties of Stimulated Cells

At first sight it may seem of little practical importance to be able to distinguish between slow progression through the G_1 phase and periods of arrest or rest. However, the factors controlling the rate of proliferation may well depend on the initial state of the cell. Quiescent, non-stimulated lymphocytes are a putative G_0 population, and Darzynkiewicz et al. (1979) have recently provided important evidence that chromatin packing of G_0 cells is more condensed than that in G_1 cells. On the basis of the difference in the extent of denatured DNA after acid treatment, it has been possible to distinguish between G_0 and G_1 lymphocytes. Farber and Baserga (1969) also provided evidence that cells originating from a putative G_0 compartment were biochemically distinct from those cells actively progressing through the division sequence. They found that whilst hydroxyurea killed DNA-synthesising cells in a variety of continually renewing populations, it was ineffective in inflicting any lethal damage upon hepatocytes which had been stimulated into DNA synthesis by partial hepatectomy. Figure 7 illustrates the effect of two S-phase-specific cytotoxic drugs upon the DNA synthesising cell populations of the mouse jejunal crypt and the mouse seminal vesicle.

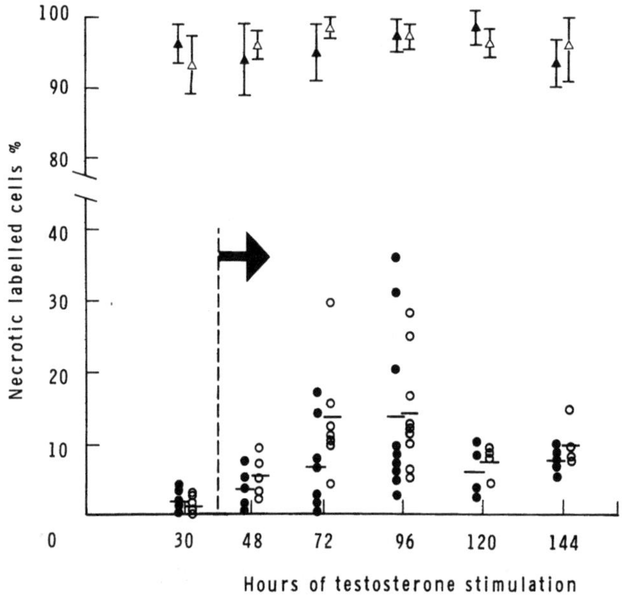

Fig. 7. Changes in the susceptibility of DNA-synthesising cells from the jejunum (*triangles*) and seminal vesicle (*circles*) to either cytosine arabinoside (*closed symbols*) or hydroxyurea (*open symbols*). Daily treatment with 250 μg testosterone propionate began at 14 days after castration. All mice received injections of 25 μCi ^{3}H-thymidine and, 0.5 h later, either cytosine arabinoside (400 mg/kg body weight) or hydroxyurea (1,500 mg/kg body weight). All mice were killed 3.5 h after ^{3}H-thymidine injection, and 1,000 cells were counted for each animal. Each *symbol* denotes investigation of a single animal; results for the jejunum are given as mean ± standard deviation. Mice killed at the time intervals to the *right* of the *vertical dashed line* have seminal vesicles largely composed of newly born epithelial cells. Continuous ^{3}H-thymidine labelling has indicated that all the original G_0 population has entered DNA synthesis before 40 h of testosterone treatment (Alison and Wright 1979a)

Intestinal crypt cells largely make unimpeded progress from one mitotic division to another without entering G_0 (Fig. 5), and the cells in DNA synthesis are highly susceptible to the lethal effects of both agents (see Fig. 8a). In marked contrast, few stimulated seminal vesicle cells in DNA synthesis succumb to such lethal effects (see Fig. 8b), although this resistance appears to diminish in those cells recently born by mitotic division. These data may be of significance to the regulation of cell proliferation, suggesting that the mechanisms involved in the transition of cells from G_1 to S may be quite different from those involved in a G_0 to S transition. These conclusions are reinforced by the fact that the differential effect was not restricted to a large dose of just one drug. Cytosine arabinoside is a DNA polymerase inhibitor, whilst hydroxyurea is a ribonucleotide reductase inhibitor. In addition, cytosine arabinoside and hydroxyurea caused a 6- to 8-h inhibition of DNA synthesis in both the crypt cells and the stimulated seminal vesicle cells.

It appears that the proliferative rate of rodent prostatic tissues is slow because most cells are in a unique physiological state, a phase of proliferative rest termed G_0. However, the processes involved in retrieving these cells need bear no relationship to the continued progression of cells through the division sequence.

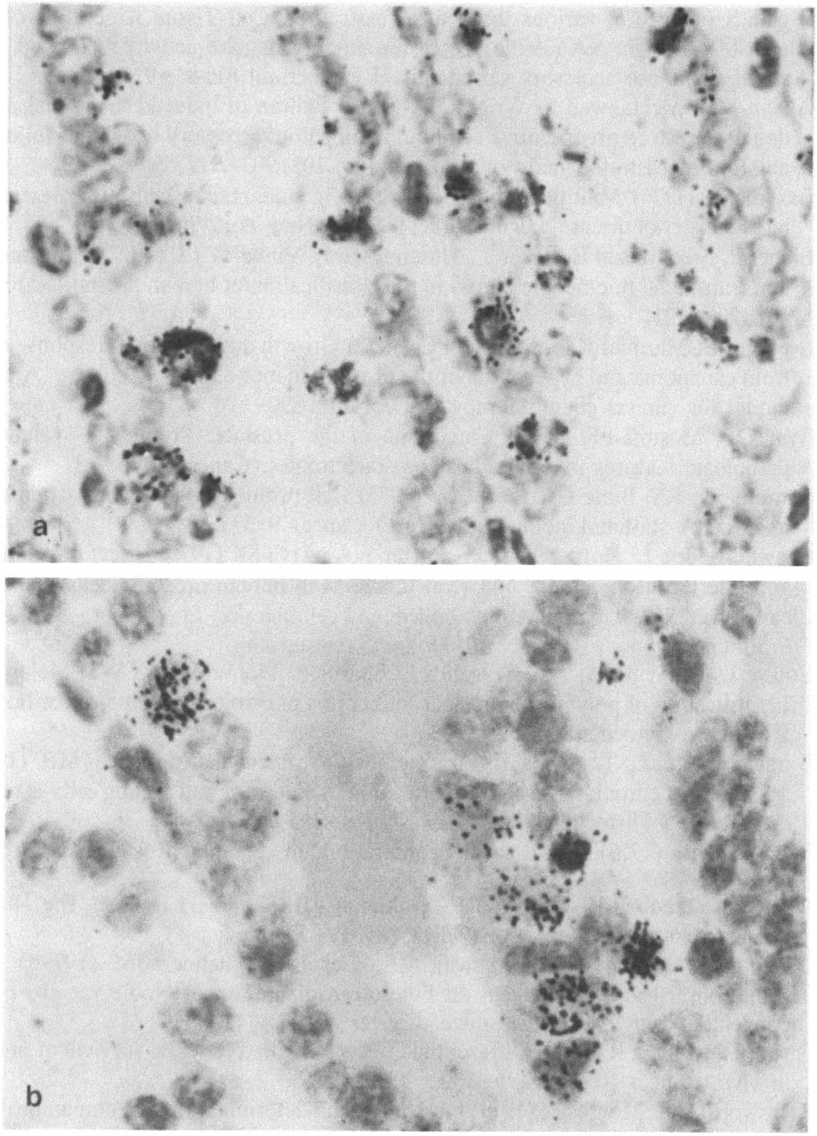

Fig. 8a, b. Autoradiographs of jejunal crypt cells (**a**) and seminal vesicle cells (**b**) following injection of ^{3}H-thymidine and cytosine arabinoside (see legend to Fig. 7) after 72 h of testosterone treatment. Most labelled cells in the jejunum were necrotic, whilst most of the labelled cells in the seminal vesicle appeared normal. H and E, 1,300×

5 References

Aherne WA, Camplejohn RS, Wright NA (1977) An introduction to cell population kinetics. Edward Arnold, London, pp 11–14

Ahmed K, Wilson MJ (1978) Chromatin controls in the prostate. In: Busch H (ed) The cell nucleus, vol 6. Academic Press, New York, pp 409–459

Alison MR, Wright NA (1979a) Testosterone-induced cell proliferation in the accessory sex glands of mice at various times after castration. Cell Tissue Kinet 12: 461–475

Alison MR, Wright NA (1979b) Testosterone 5α-reductase activity as related to proliferative status in mouse accessory sex glands. J Endocrinol 81: 83–92

Alison MR, McHanwell S, Wright NA (1979) Failure of induced functional activity and cell deficit to restore preoperative cell number in paired accessory sex glands following unilateral ablation in castrated male mice. Anat Rec 193: 903–912

Baserga R (1976) Multiplication and division in mammalian cells. In: Baserga R (ed) The biochemistry of disease, vol 6. Marcel Dekker, New York, pp 349–360

Bichel P, Frederiksen P, Kjaer T, Thommesen P, Vindelov LL (1977) Flow microfluorometry and transrectal fine-needle biopsy in the classification of human prostatic carcinoma. Cancer 40: 1206–1211

Brehmer B, Marquardt H, Madsen PO (1972) Growth and hormonal response of cells derived from carcinoma and hyperplasia of the prostate in monolayer cell culture. A possible in vitro model for clinical chemotherapy. J Urol 108: 890–896

Byar DP, Mostofi FK (1972) Carcinoma of the prostate: Prognostic evaluation of certain pathologic features in 208 radical prostatectomies. Cancer 30: 5–13

Camplejohn RS, Bone G, Aherne W (1973) Cell proliferation in rectal carcinoma and rectal mucosa. A stathmokinetic study. Eur J Cancer 9: 577–581

Chawda R, Job L, Horoszewicz JS, Carter WA, Arya SK (1979) Effect of bromodeoxyuridine and interferon on cellular and viral functions in human prostatic cells. Oncology 36:35–39

Cleaver JE (1967) Thymidine metabolism and cell kinetics. In: Neuberger A, Tatum EL (eds) Frontiers of biology, vol 6. North-Holland, Amsterdam

Collste L, Darzynkiewicz Z, Traganos F, Sharpless TK, Whitmore WF, Melamed MR (1979) Identification of polymorphonuclear leukocytes in cytological samples for flow cytometry. J Histochem Cytochem 27: 390–393

Darzynkiewicz Z, Traganos F, Andreef M, Sharpless T, Melamed MR (1979) Different sensitivity of chromatin to acid denaturation in quiescent and cycling cells as revealed by flow cytometry. J Histochem Cytochem 27: 478–485

Dermer GB (1978) Basal cell proliferation in benign prostatic hyperplasia. Cancer 41: 1857–1862

Drago JR, Ikeda RM, Maurer RE, Goldman LB, Tesluk H (1979a) The Nb rat: Prostatic adenocarcinoma model. Invest Urol 16: 353–359

Drago JR, Maurer RE, Gershwin ME, Eckels D, Palmer JM (1979b) The effect of 5-fluorouracil and adriamycin on heterotransplantation of Noble rat prostatic tumours in congenitally athymic (nude) mice. Cancer 44: 424–430

Farber E, Baserga R (1969) Differential effects of hydroxyurea on survival of proliferating cells in vivo. Cancer Res 29: 136–139

Farnsworth WE, Montes M (1979) Derivation and determination of a human prostatic epithelial index. Arch Androl 2: 85–88

Frederiksen P, Thommesen P, Kjaer TB, Bichel P (1978) Flow cytometric DNA analysis in fine needle aspiration biopsies from patients with prostatic lesions. Diagnostic value and relation to clinical stages. Acta Pathol Microbiol Scand [A] 86: 461–464

Fulker MJ, Cooper EH, Tanaka T (1971) Proliferation and ultrastructure of papillary transitional cell carcinoma of the human bladder. Cancer 27: 71–82

Hamburger AW, Salmon SE (1977) Primary bioassay of human tumour stem cells. Science 197: 461–463

Hamburger AW, Salmon SE, Kim MB, Trent JM, Soehnlen BJ, Alberts DS, Schmidt HJ (1978) Direct cloning of human ovarian carcinoma cells in agar. Cancer Res 38: 3438–3444

Helpap B, Stiens R (1975) The cell proliferation of epithelial metaplasia in the prostate gland. Virchows Arch [Cell Pathol] 19: 69–76

Helpap B, Stiens R, Bruhl P (1974) Autoradiographic in vitro investigations on prostatic tissue with the C-14- and H-3-thymidine double-labelling method. Beitr Pathol Anat Allgem Pathol 151: 65–74

Hindsley JP, Fried FA, Avis I, Avis FP (1978) Transplantation of human prostate neoplasia into the nude mouse. In: Bonney WW (ed) Workshop on genitourinary cancer immunology. Natl Cancer Inst Monogr 49: 67–69

Isaacs JT, Heston WDW, Weissman RM, Coffey DS (1978) Animal models of hormone-sensitive and -insensitive prostatic adenocarcinomas, Dunning R-3327-H, R-3327-HI, and R-3327-AT. Cancer Res 38: 4353–4359

King RJB, Mainwaring WIP (1974) Steroid-cell interactions. Butterworths, London, pp 56–85

Lasnitzki I, Whitaker RH, Withycombe JFR (1975) The effect of steroid hormones on the growth pattern and RNA synthesis in human benign prostatic hyperplasia in organ culture. Br J Cancer 32: 168–178

Liavag I (1968) Mitotic activity of prostatic epithelium. Acta Pathol Microbiol Scand 73: 19–28

Mainwaring WIP (1977) The mechanism of action of androgens. Springer, New York (Monographs on endocrinology, vol 10)

McMahon MJ, Butler AVJ, Thomas GH (1972) Morphological responses of prostatic carcinoma to testosterone in organ culture. Br J Cancer 26: 388–394

McMahon MJ, Thomas GH (1973) Morphological changes of benign prostatic hyperplasia in culture. Br J Cancer 27: 323–335

McRae CU, Ghanadian R, Fotherby K, Chisholm GD (1973) The effect of testosterone on the human prostate in organ culture. Br J Urol 45: 156–162

Muntzing J, Liljekvist J, Murphy GP (1979) Chalones and stroma as possible growth-limiting factors in the rat ventral prostate. Invest Urol 16: 399–394

Pollard M (1973) Spontaneous prostate adenocarcinomas in aged germ-free Wistar rats. J Natl Cancer Inst 51: 1235–1241

Rao BR, Nakeff A, Eaton C, Heston WDW (1978) Establishment and characterisation of an in vitro clonogenic cell assay for the R-3327-At Copenhagen rat prostatic tumor. Cancer Res 38: 4431–4439

Shain SA, McCullough B, Nitchuk WM (1979) Primary and transplantable adenocarcinomas of the AxC rat ventral prostate gland: Morphologic characterisation and estimation of C_{19}-steroid metabolism by early-passage tumours. J Natl Cancer Inst 62: 313–322

Shipman PAM, Littlewood V, Riches AC, Thomas GH (1975) Differences in proliferative activity of rat and human prostate in culture. Br J Cancer 31: 570–580

Spooner ME, Cooper EH (1972) Chromosome constitution of transitional-cell carcinoma of the urinary bladder. Cancer 29: 1401–1412

Sprenger E, Witte S (1979) The diagnostic significance of nuclear deoxyribonucleic acid measurement in automated cytology. J Histochem Cytochem 27: 520–521

Spriggs AI (1976) Chromosomes in human neoplastic diseases. In: Symington T, Carter RL (eds) Scientific foundations of oncology. Heinemann, London, pp 147–155

Stiens R, Helpap B, Bruhl P (1975) The proliferation of prostatic epithelium in chronic prostatitis. Urol Res 3: 21–24

Steel GG (1977) Growth kinetics of tumours. University Press, Oxford

Timms BG, Chandler JA, Sinowatz F (1976) The ultrastructure of basal cells of rat and dog prostate. Cell Tissue Res 173: 543–554

Tuohimaa P, Niemi M (1968) The effect of testosterone on cell renewal and mitotic cycles in sex accessory glands of castrated mice. Acta Endocrinol (Kbh) 58: 696–703

Weissman RM, Coffey DS, Scott WW (1977) Cell kinetic studies of prostatic cancer: adjuvant therapy in animal models. Oncology 34: 133–137

Wimber DE (1963) Methods for studying cell proliferation with emphasis on DNA labels. In: Lamerton LF, Fry RJM (eds) Cell proliferation. Blackwells, Oxford, pp 1–17

Zetterberg A, Esposti PL (1976) Cytophotometric DNA-analysis of aspirated cells from prostatic carcinoma. Acta Cytol 20: 46–57

Hormonal Relationships, Receptors, and Tumour Markers

M. E. Harper, P. Chaisiri, J. Slade, W. B. Peeling, and K. Griffiths*

Tenovus Institute for Cancer Research, Welsh National School of Medicine,
GB – Cardiff CF4 4XN

1 Introduction

Prostatic cancer is one of the most common causes of death from malignant disease in men. It is unfortunate, however, that this particular form of cancer and benign hyperplasia of the prostate gland are generally considered mere appurtenances of advancing years and relatively little research has been directed to the study of the biological factors that may be concerned with the aetiology of the condition. Furthermore, prostatic cancer is often clinically recognised only when the disease has become systemic and has extended beyond the prostate, yet there is little information on potential risk factors relating to the disease, and limited data on the practical value of various 'tumour markers' for the early detection of the condition.

Although the classic laboratory experiments of Dr. Charles Huggins and his colleagues (Huggins and Clark 1940; Huggins and Hodges 1941; Huggins et al. 1941) clearly established the androgen dependence of the prostatic cancer cell, thereby laying the foundation for treatment of the disease by oestrogen or antiandrogen therapy, the endocrine factors concerned with the aetiology of cancer of the prostate are little understood. There is, as yet, no evidence that hormones can initiate prostatic cancer, although the disease has not been reported in a prepubertally castrated male and it would seem that any role for hormones in the pathogenesis of this condition is essentially permissive.

It is not surprising, however, that investigations into the 'risk factors' concerned with such a hormone-dependent cancer, were directed primarily to a search for an endocrine 'abnormality' of the prostatic cancer patient, although at present there is little evidence that a changed endocrine status is implicated in the promotion of neoplasia (Griffiths et al. 1979). It is interesting, however, that although zones of the true prostate undergo a progressive, but slow atrophy with age (McNeal 1975), certain older men have prostatic tissue showing glandular morphology comparable to that seen in glands from younger men. Furthermore, McNeal (1970, 1972) has described an age-related increase in atypical hyperplasia of the prostate, changes which were considered premalignant and which related closely to prostatic carcinoma. Whether this age-related hyperplasia reflects some degree of hormonal stimulation associated with a change in the endocrine status of the male remains to be determined.

Also relevant in this context is the presence of small foci of latent, asymptomatic, differentiated carcinoma in the prostate of the older man. Although a common finding

* The authors wish to thank Tenovus Organisation for their generous financial support

Recent Results in Cancer Research, Vol. 78
© Springer-Verlag Berlin · Heidelberg 1981

in the peripheral zone of the prostate gland, it is believed that many of these microscopic foci of cancer never become clinically evident (Varkarakis et al. 1970; Correa et al. 1974). The time course of development of such latent carcinoma is not known, although there is evidence that a time lapse of at least 20 years could occur between the appearance of neoplasia and the clinical manifestation of the disease (Hirst and Bergman 1954). The relationship between the changing endocrine status with ageing and these microcarcinoma may be of particular interest. It is also noteworthy that despite the low incidence of carcinoma of the prostate in Japan, latent carcinoma is as prevalent there as in a Caucasian population (Buell and Dunn 1965; Haenszel and Kurihara 1968), and investigations exploring the possibility of a different endocrine status in the ageing Japanese male could well be of immense value in helping us to understand the biological factors concerned in the promotion of prostatic cancer.

2 Hormonal Status

Figure 1 provides some indication of the hormones and glands that could be concerned in controlling the growth and function of the prostate gland. Testosterone, synthesised and secreted by the testis, is considered the principal plasma androgen although other C_{19}-steroids, dehydroepiandrosterone (DHA) and its sulphate, together with androstenedione are secreted in relatively high concentrations from the adrenal gland and contribute to the androgenic status of the male. These adrenal androgens could be metabolised by the prostate to more potent androgens (Pike et al. 1970; Harper et al. 1974).

Studies by Vermeulen et al. (1972) have suggested that the plasma concentration of testosterone tends to fall after the sixth decade, although the testis and adrenal can still respond to trophic hormone stimulation despite ageing (Doerr and Pirke 1974; Kley et al. 1975). The concentration of oestradiol-17β in the plasma increases with age (Pirke and Doerr 1973; Kley et al. 1974). Oestradiol-17β is secreted by the testis (Longcope et al. 1972) and, furthermore, is synthesised from the peripheral metabolism of the adrenal C_{19}-steroid, androstenedione; it is this increased peripheral aromatisation of androstenedione that is believed responsible for the higher levels of oestradiol-17β in the older man (Longcope et al. 1969; MacDonald et al. 1972).

It is equally important to consider the level of sex hormone-binding globulin (SHBG) in plasma. Little of the testosterone in plasma is free and unbound to protein, but it is this free hormone which is considered the biologically active material that can be transferred into the cells of the prostate gland. The level of SHBG also increases with age (Vermeulen et al. 1971), which will therefore influence the amount of hormone taken up by the target tissues. Prolactin, which appears to have a synergistic role with luteinising hormone (LH) in controlling the secretory activity of testis, might also influence not only the uptake of testosterone by the prostate, but the biological effect of other protein hormones, such as growth hormone, on the gland. A recent review (Griffiths et al. 1979) discusses in detail the endocrinology of prostatic disease. It was reasonable, however, that studies directed to understanding the endocrinology of prostatic disease should be concentrated on the determination of plasma hormone levels of patients with the condition. Unfortunately, the accumulated data have tended to be disappointing (Harper et al. 1976; Bartsch et al. 1977; Hammond et al. 1977).

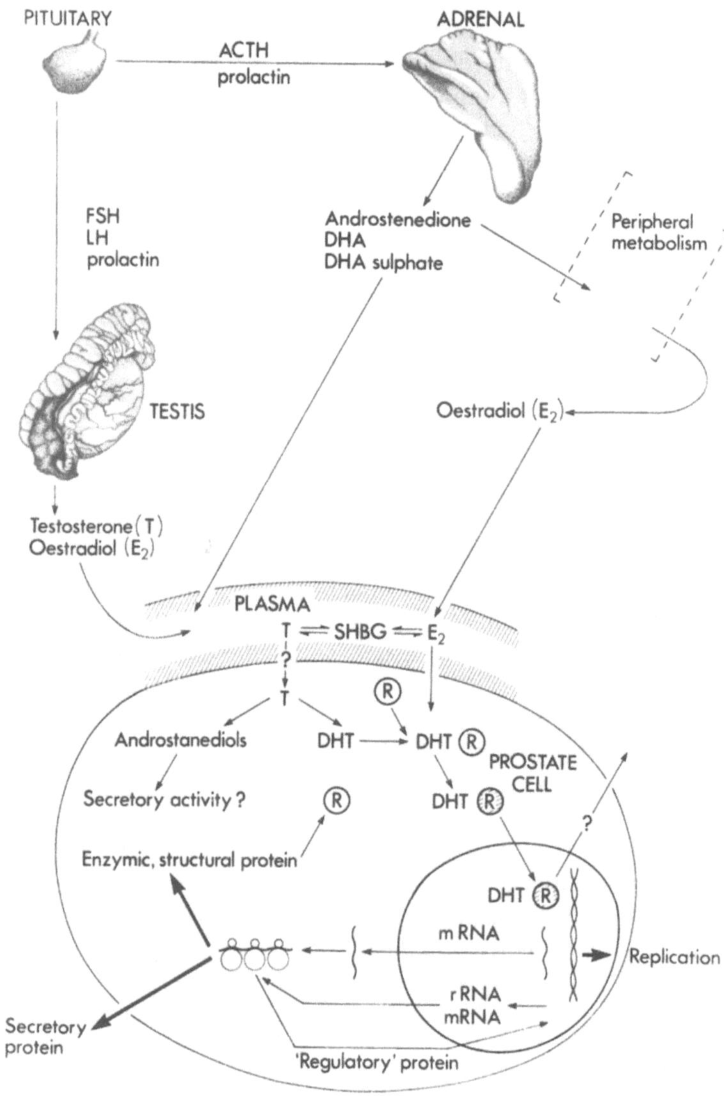

Fig. 1. Schematic representation of certain aspects of the endocrinology relating to control of the prostate gland. *DHA*, dehydroepiandrosterone; *DHT*, 5α-dihydrotestosterone; *SHBG*, sex hormone-binding globulin; *R*, specific intracellular receptor; *DHT-R*, steroid-receptor complex; *mRNA* and *rRNA*, messenger and ribosomal ribonucleic acid, respectively. *Question marks* refer to processes not completely elucidated

A detailed study in the United Kingdom, undertaken by the British Prostate Study Group (1979), was focussed on the relationship between hormone concentrations in plasma of patients with proven prostatic cancer and various clinical parameters. There were no differences between hormone levels of patients with cancer and the controls. Moreover, there was no systematic change in the group means of the hormone concentrations related to the progression of the disease from stage T0 to stage T4 (Table 1). Wide variations in hormone concentrations were found, levels in older men

Table 1. Plasma hormone concentrations of patients with prostatic carcinoma grouped according to (a) UICC classification of primary tumours and (b) metastatic spread

		Age (years)	Plasma hormone concentrations					
			LH mIU/ml	FSH mIU/ml	GH μU/ml	Prolactin mμ/ml	T ng/ml	E_2 pg/ml
(a) Primary tumour								
T0 category	Mean	71	6.4	15.5	3.1	0.1	4.5	29.5
(*n* = 24)	SD	9.04	5.33	14.05	3.72	0.13	1.48	17.65
T1 category	Mean	68	6.7	16.9	1.6	0.1	4.6	27.0
(*n* = 14)	SD	7.07	5.28	16.07	2.44	0.09	2.03	9.33
T2 category	Mean	71	5.4	15.1	3.8	0.1	4.4	29.4
(*n* = 31)	SD	9.23	4.13	14.03	7.06	0.10	1.60	11.06
T3 category	Mean	70	8.2	16.8	2.5	0.1	4.1	26.2
(*n* = 73)	SD	7.86	8.09	17.27	3.49	0.11	1.53	12.11
T4 category	Mean	68	6.5	14.6	3.7	0.1	3.7	24.5
(*n* = 21)	SD	7.43	7.15	22.46	4.85	0.11	1.31	7.53
(b) Metastatic spread								
Patients without metastases M0	Mean	70	7.8	18.5	2.4	0.10	4.3	25.9
(*n* = 78)	SD	8.15	7.80	19.70	2.71	0.11	1.38	9.46
Patients with metastases M1	Mean	70	6.0	13.0	3.4	0.10	4.1	27.1
(*n* = 72)	SD	8.28	5.05	13.00	4.28	0.12	1.74	13.24

T, testosterone; E_2, oestradiol-17β; *n*, numbers of patients; SD, standard deviation; *NS*, not significant

in their seventies being similar to those of young men. Generally the hormone concentrations appeared unrelated to the presence of metastatic disease, although when the data were subjected to multivariate analysis it was seen that growth hormone concentration was a major contributory factor in the discrimination between patients with (M1) and without (M0) metastases. The study emphasised the potential value of multivariate analysis in assessment of the complex endocrine status of the ageing male in relation to disease. Analysis of the preliminary hormone and clinical data clearly indicated that group differences existed when the computer print-outs were considered (Fig. 2), although the clinical relevance of the higher growth hormone levels in patients with metastatic disease is obviously not clear.

Promotion of prostatic neoplasia may well be dependent on some particular, abnormal endocrine status of certain individuals, but current evidence indicates therefore that it will be very difficult to identify a high-risk group from simple plasma analysis of hormones.

It is possible, however, that the recent development by the Tenovus Institute of radio-immunoassays for salivary steroids (Walker et al. 1978a, 1979; Turkes et al. 1979; Fahmy et al. 1980) might allow a more detailed study of the chrono-endocrinology relating to ageing and prostatic cancer. The non-invasive nature of saliva collection makes sequential sampling very easy and the fact that the salivary steroid concentration reflects the level of non-protein-bound, free, biologically active steroid in plasma renders the assays of immense value. Recent studies of testosterone levels in saliva (Walker et al. 1980) from a group of males clearly demonstrate their potential and illustrate the ease with which the circadian rhythm of testosterone production can be shown (Fig. 3).

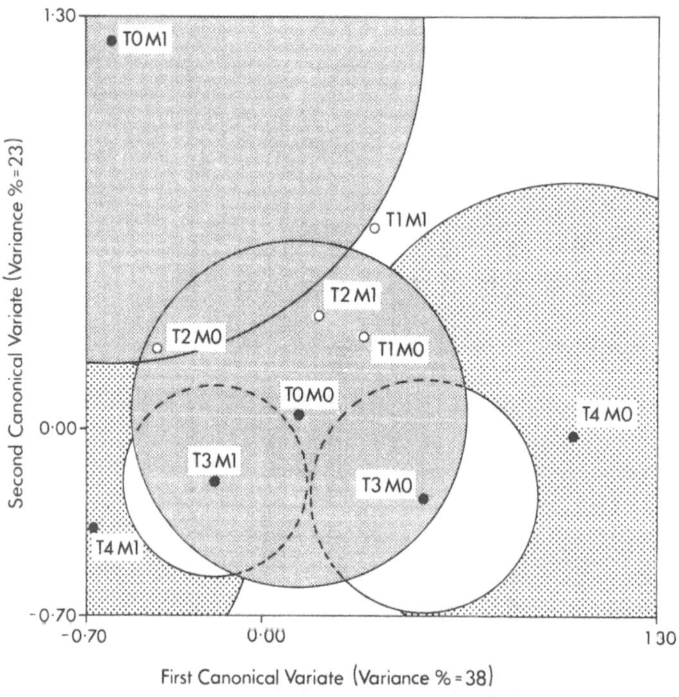

Fig. 2. Multivariate analysis of data on hormone concentrations and patients age, showing group separation based on stage (*T*) and metastatic status (*M*)

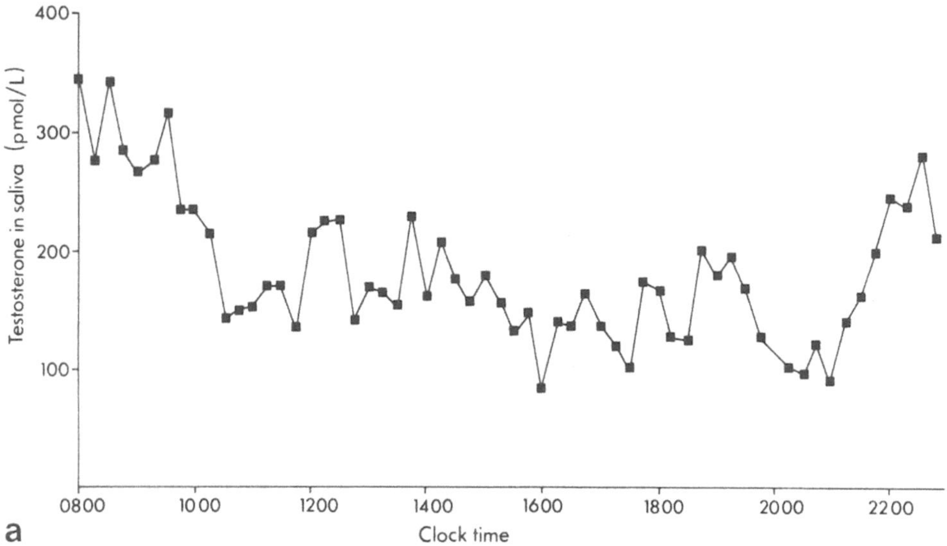

a

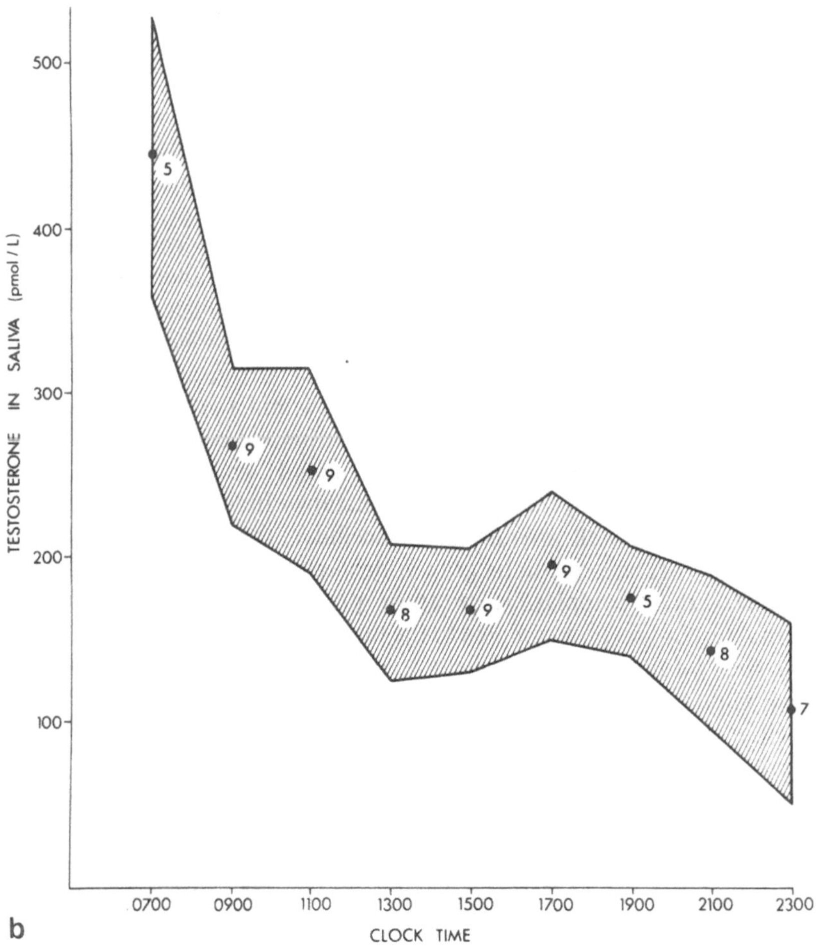

b

Fig. 3a, b. Circadian rhythm in salivary testosterone from one individual (**a**) and a group of males (**b**). Numbers refer to subjects

It may be, however, that the most appropriate time to study hormone profiles is earlier in life, before the disease is clinically manifest. It was always hoped that factors that might reflect the hormonal status of younger men prior to cancer development – demographic features such as marital status, sex drive and other social and hormonal influences in the early life of men who present with prostatic cancer – might help to differentiate a high-risk group, but such studies have generally been disappointing (King et al. 1963; Steele et al. 1971; Greenwald et al. 1974). The close correlation between the incidence of prostatic cancer and carcinoma of the breast in various countries around the world (Wynder et al. 1971), and the established relationship between early first-term birth and risk of developing breast cancer (MacMahon et al. 1970) possibly suggest that various biological changes in adolescence may 'trigger' biochemical events, which in later life are manifest in neoplastic growth. In relation to this, a recent investigation (Rotkin 1977) suggested that delayed onset of sexuality in the late adolescent period, with an early suppression of sexual activity, were features prevalent in those with prostatic cancer.

2.1 Role of Testosterone in Androgen Receptor Assays

Consideration must also be given to the possibility that biochemical changes within the prostatic cells might be responsible for an increased responsiveness to normal hormone levels in plasma. Man and dog are virtually alone in the animal kingdom in their susceptability to prostatic hyperplasia, and the epithelial tissue of the peripheral zone of the human prostate is the predominant site of origin of carcinoma. The difference between this type of androgen-dependent prostatic epithelial tissue and those of other male accessory glands such as the seminal vesicles, which rarely develop cancer, remains to be determined. Particular attention is presently being devoted to the cellular processes concerned with the mode of action of testosterone (Fig. 1). It is now well established that testosterone is metabolised within the prostatic cell to 5α-dihydrotestosterone, which is the active androgen within the cell (see Griffiths et al. 1979), although other metabolites, the 5α-androstanediols, may also have specific biochemical roles in the control of prostatic function. Indeed the pattern of testosterone metabolism may well provide an intracellular, regulatory process. The 5α-dihydrotestosterone regulates prostatic growth through a mechanism involving its specific association with a cytoplasmic receptor protein (Fig. 1), followed by translocation of the steroid-receptor complex to the nucleus. Binding of the complex to nuclear acceptor sites on the chromatin elicits transcription, mRNA synthesis, and tissue growth. It is important to determine whether receptor characteristics in diseased prostatic tissue differ from those of normal tissue (Davies 1978) in such a way that the affinity of the protein for 5α-dihydrotestosterone, or possibly other metabolites of testosterone or oestradiol-17β, could influence prostatic growth. Furthermore, since it has been shown that the analysis of oestradiol-17β receptor protein content in breast tumour tissue can be used to predict the response to endocrine therapy of patients with advanced cancer (McGuire et al. 1975), it has been hoped that 5α-dihydrotestosterone receptor levels in prostatic carcinoma could also be of value in determining the most appropriate form of therapy. It is well accepted now that breast tumours devoid of oestradiol receptors are rarely influenced by endocrine therapy.

The value of androgen receptor assays in human prostatic carcinoma as a predictor of endocrine response has not yet been established, however. Although the methodology is now available to study these relatively labile proteins (Davies et al. 1977; Shain and Boesel 1978), obviously the nature of the tumour tissue available for analysis is important in determining the real value of the receptor status of the tissue in relation to response to therapy. The material obtained by electroresection is clearly unacceptable. Analysis of metastatic deposits could well be the most useful, although such tissue is difficult to obtain. A recent report by Ekman et al. (1979), who analysed tissue removed by perineal punch needle biopsy of primary tumour (50–200 mg tissue), indicated that reliable receptor data could be obtained which related well to short-term response to endocrine therapy. Although support for this work has been provided by the work of Mobbs et al. (1978), who measured androgen receptor content by means of a protamine sulphate precipitation assay, de Voogt and Dingjan (1978), with an agar gel electrophoretic procedure, were unable to relate receptor levels to response. Clearly further studies are necessary in this important field to establish the clinical value of the oestrogen receptor concentration in prostatic cancer.

3 Some Aspects of Tumour Marker Analysis

3.1 Polyamines

The high concentration of aliphatic polyamines in prostatic tissue and in seminal plasma is well documented (Williams-Ashman et al. 1972a, 1975), although their role in human reproduction is uncertain. Polyamines, however, influence micromolecular synthesis in prostatic tissue preparations (Williams-Ashman et al. 1972a), effect RNA transcription, and give rise to the increased spermidine levels in proliferating neoplastic tissue (Snyder and Russell 1970); the related activity of ornithine-decarboxylase, an enzyme concerned with polyamine synthesis, indicates an association with DNA replication (Williams-Ashman et al. 1972b). It was reasonable to expect that patients with malignant tumours might have elevated levels of polyamines in urine and plasma, and high levels have been reported in such patients (Russell 1978; Marton et al. 1973). The possibility existed, therefore, that measurement of polyamine levels in plasma might reflect normal growth patterns within prostatic tissue. The studies of Russell et al. (1978) provided considerable support for this concept, and it seemed that polyamine analysis might offer a valuable tumour marker for the early detection of prostatic carcinoma. It has generally been accepted, however, that methods for the measurement of polyamines in biological fluids are tedious, and/or lack sensitivity. To assess the value of polyamine analysis, both in the diagnosis of early cancer and in the assessment of response to therapy, it was necessary to develop sensitive and relatively rapid radio-immunoassays for the specific analysis of spermine and spermidine. These assays have been previously described (Chaisiri et al. 1979, 1980) and some of the preliminary data from patients with prostatic disease are shown in the following section.

Table 2 shows the mean ± standard deviation and ranges of spermine concentration in the plasma of patients with benign prostatic hyperplasia and prostatic carcinoma compared with normal male subjects. There were no significant differences between the groups, and of the 54 patients with carcinoma only three had spermine levels higher than the normal range. When the primary prostatic tumours were classified into

Table 2. Levels of plasma spermine in patients with prostatic tumours and in normal subjects

	Age (years)	No. of subjects	Spermine (pmol/ml)		No. with elevated levels[a]
			Mean ± SD	Range	
(A) Benign	52–82	20	210 ± 140	50–540	2
Malignant	48–89	54	210 ± 110	60–640	3
Normal males	18–79	66	200 ± 100	50–320	
(B) Patients with malignant tumour staged by UICC T categories					
T0		8	200 ± 90	70–380	
T1		6	200 ± 60	120–270	
T2		12	210 ± 80	100–390	
T3		18	210 ± 120	130–640	
T4		9	240 ± 160	60–520	
(C) Patients with and without metastases					
M0		24	230 ± 80	130–520	
M1		19	230 ± 150	20–640	

[a] Elevated level is defined as a higher level than the mean + 2 SD for normal males

Table 3. Levels of plasma spermidine in patients with prostate tumours and in normal subjects

	Age (years)	No. of subjects	Spermidine (pmol/ml)		No. with elevated levels[a]
			Mean ± SD	Range	
(A) Benign	52–85	40	198 ± 169	36– 705	3
Malignant	49–93	52	316 ± 240	36–1,015[b]	13
Normal males	19–79	61	200 ± 137	48– 636	
(B) Patients with malignant tumour staged by UICC T categories					
T0		14	305 ± 228	99– 912	3
T1		9	305 ± 237	43– 826	2
T2		13	374 ± 294	36–1,015	4
T3		8	225 ± 105	108– 437	0
T4		5	400 ± 280	159– 826	2
(C) Patients with and without metastases					
M0		21	285 ± 202	36– 826	4
M1		15	304 ± 192	117– 791	3

[a] Elevated level is defined as a higher level than the mean + 2 SD for normal males
[b] Difference from normal males in statistically significant (2 p = 0.001)

T categories according to the UICC system (Wallace et al. 1975) and the metastatic status was noted as M0 and M1, again, there was no correlation between spermine concentration and clinical staging or between those with localised cancer and those with widespread metastatic disease. Spermine concentration in plasma therefore appears to be of little value, either for detection or in monitoring response to therapy.

Table 3 shows similar data for spermidine concentrations in the plasma of patients with prostatic disease. Although the mean spermidine concentration in the plasma of patients with prostatic cancer was significantly higher than that of normal males, only 13 of the 52 patients had values 2SD above the normal. Three of the 40 patients with benign prostatic hyperplasia had elevated levels. Again, spermidine levels did not relate to primary tumour staging or to metastatic status of the patient. It should be noted however that it has been suggested that spermidine is present in plasma predominantly in the conjugated form (Rosenblum et al. 1978), and the radio-immunoassay used in the Institute measures only free spermidine.

The higher levels of spermidine in certain samples of plasma from patients with prostate cancer are to some extent in agreement with previous results (Sanford et al. 1975; Fair et al. 1975; Lipton et al. 1976), which indicated that urinary polyamine concentrations were elevated in 70% of such patients. The number of patients was smaller in these studies, however, and the quoted elevations were not 2SD higher than

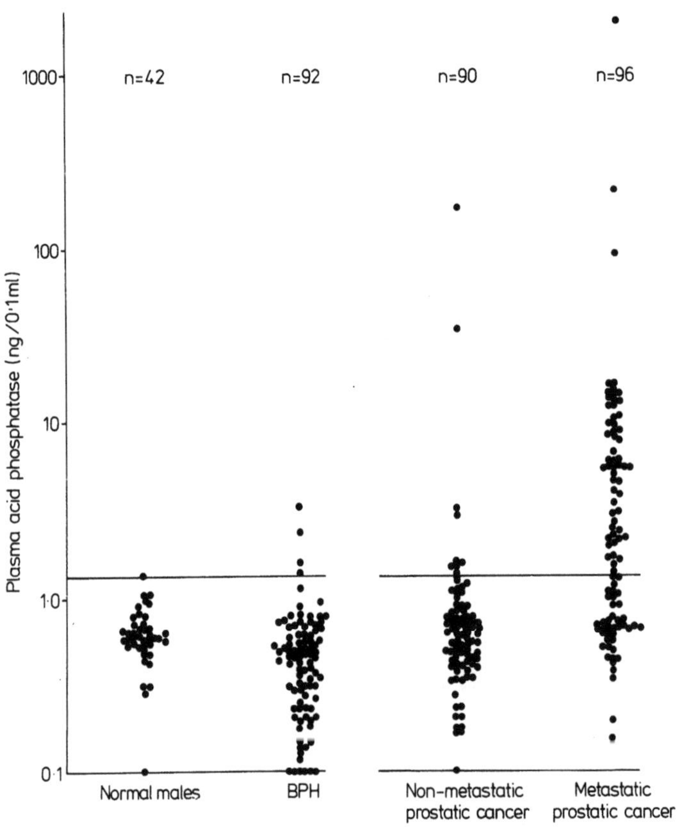

Fig. 4. Plasma acid phosphatase levels in BPH, non-metastatic prostate cancer, and metastatic prostate cancer, compared with those in a control group of normal males

the mean concentration for normal males. Total spermidine concentration is also measured by the urinary assay.

3.2 Acid Phosphatase

One of the first tumour markers to be measured in serum was the activity of the enzyme acid phosphatase. This enzyme is secreted by prostatic epithelium and although its physiological role is not clear, it has been established for some time (Gutman and Gutman 1938; Huggins and Hodges 1941) that serum acid phosphatase activity is elevated in patients with prostatic carcinoma, 65%–90% of patients with bone metastases, and 5%–10% of those with clinically demonstrable metastatic cancer (Yam 1974). Serum acid phosphatase activity can, however, be attributed to many tissues other than the prostate. The tissue specificity of this marker is therefore to some extent limited unless the 'prostatic proportion' of the activity is defined. The isolation of tissue isoenzymes and the use of particular enzymatic incubation conditions and specific inhibitors, together with the incorporation of certain enzyme substrates, was found to be unsatisfactory; the realisation that the enzyme activity was

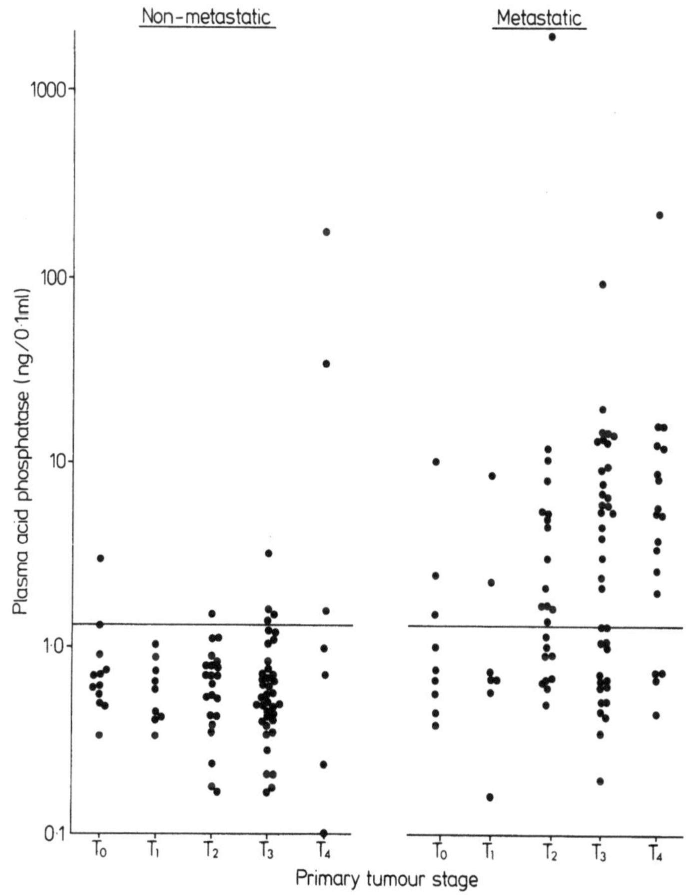

Fig. 5. Plasma acid phosphatase levels in non-metastatic and metastatic prostate cancer in relation to stage classification

to some extent irrelevant to the role of the enzyme as a tumour marker stimulated the development of an immunoassay for the measurement of the enzyme protein.
Initial reports of studies with antisera raised to purified prostatic acid phosphatase were encouraging, with an increased sensitivity being found for the detection of elevated levels of the protein in earlier stages of prostatic cancer (Foti et al. 1977; Chu et al. 1977/1978; Romas et al. 1979). The involvement of the Institute in the British Prostate Study Group's hormonal survey of patients presenting with cancer stimulated the search for effective tumour markers and a radio-immunoassay for prostatic acid phosphatase had been established, together with those for carcinoembryonic antigen (CEA) and β-hCG. Since samples of plasma from various clinics were frozen and sent to the Institute for analysis, obviously the immunoassay for the protein offered more stability than an assay determining enzyme activity.
Very briefly, the enzyme was purified from benign hyperplastic tissue by ammonium sulphate precipitation, followed by DEAE cellulose and Sephadex G 150 column chromatography. The enzyme was homogeneous in polyacrylamide gel electrophoresis, and antisera were raised to the protein in New Zealand white rabbits. A double-antibody assay with ^{125}I-labelled antigen was established. Although certain investigators (Vihko et al. 1978) have been able to show a complete separation of the cancer group with elevated serum enzyme levels from the control group, Fig. 4 indicates that in this particular study, now reported, considerable overlap was found, although a larger proportion of patients with metastatic disease had higher levels. Figure 5 illustrates the data in relation to T classification. Further work is obviously required, but it is clear that progress is being made in the establishment and assessment of new assays for tumour markers.

4 References

Bartsch W, Horst HJ, Becker H, Nehse G (1977) Sex hormone binding globulin capacity, testosterone 5α-dihydrotestosterone, oestradiol and prolactin in plasma of patients with prostatic carcinoma under various types of hormonal treatment. Acta Endocrinol (Kbh) 85:650–664

British Prostate Study Group (1979) Multivariate analysis of plasma hormone concentrations in relation to clinical staging in patients with prostatic cancer. Br J Urol 51:382–389

Buell P, Dunn JE (1965) Cancer mortality among Japanese Issei and Nissei of California. Cancer 18:656–668

Chaisiri P, Harper ME, Griffiths K (1979) Plasma spermine concentration of patients with benign and malignant tumours of the breast or prostate. Clin Chim Acta 92:273–275

Chaisiri P, Harper ME, Blamey RW, Peeling WB, Griffiths K (to be published) Plasma spermidine concentrations in patients with tumours of the breast or prostate or testis. Clin Chim Acta

Chu TM, Wang MC, Scott WW, Gibbons RP, Johnson DE, Schmidt JD, Loening SA, Prout GR, Murphy GP (1977/1978) Immunochemical detection of serum prostatic acid phosphatase. Invest Urol 15:319–323

Correa RJ, Anderson RG, Gibbons RP, Tate MJ (1974) Latent carcinoma of the prostate – why the controversy? J Urol 111:644–646

Davies P (1978) Receptors in the human prostate. In: Griffiths K, Pierrepoint CG, Neville AM (eds) Tumour markers, Determination and Clinical Significance. Sixth Tenovus Workshop. Alpha Omega Alpha, Cardiff, p 175

Davies P, Thomas P, Griffiths K (1977) Measurement of free and occupied cytoplasmic and nuclear androgen receptor sites in rat ventral prostate gland. J Endocrinol 74: 393–404
de Voogt HJ, Dingjan P (1978) Steroid receptors in human prostatic cancer. Urol Res 6: 151–155
Doerr P, Pirke KM (1974) Regulation of plasma oestrogens in normal adult males. I. Response of oestradiol, oestrone and testosterone to hCG, and fluoxymesterone administration. Acta Endocrinol (Kbh) 75: 617–624
Ekman P, Snochowski M, Zetterberg A, Hogberg B, Gustafsson J-A (1979) Steroid receptor content in human prostatic carcinoma and response to endocrine therapy. Cancer 44: 1173–1181
Fahmy DR, Walker RF, Read GF (1980) Salivary steroid assays for screening endocrine function. Postgrad Med J [Suppl 1] 56: 75–78
Fair WR, Wehner N, Brorsson U (1975) Urinary polyamine levels in the diagnosis of carcinoma of the prostate. J Urol 114: 88–92
Foti AG, Cooper JF, Herschman H, Malvaey RR (1977) Detection of prostatic cancer by solid phase radioimmunoassay of serum prostatic phosphatase. N Engl J Med 297: 1357–1361
Greenwald P, Damon A, Kirmss V, Polan AK (1974) Physical and demographic features of men before developing cancer of the prostate. J Natl Cancer Inst 53: 341–346
Griffiths K, Davies P, Harper ME, Peeling WB, Pierrepoint CG (1979) The etiology and endocrinology of prostatic cancer. In: Rose DP (ed) Endocrinology of cancer, vol II. CRC Press, Florida, pp 1–55
Gutman AB, Gutman ED (1938) An acid phosphatase occurring in the serum of patients with metastasizing carcinoma of the prostate gland. J Clin Invest 17: 473–480
Haenszel W, Kurihara M (1968) Studies of Japanese migrants. I. Mortality from cancer and other diseases among Japanese in the United States. J Natl Cancer Inst 40: 43–68
Hammond GL, Kontturi M, Määttälä P, Puukka M, Vihko R (1977) Serum FSH, LH and prolactin in normal males and patients with prostatic disease. Clin Endocrinol 7: 129–135
Harper ME, Pike A, Peeling WB, Griffiths K (1974) Steroids of adrenal origin metabolised by human prostatic tissue in vivo and in vitro. J Endocrinol 60: 117–125
Harper ME, Peeling WB, Cowley T, Brownsey BG, Phillips MEA, Groom G, Fahmy DR, Griffiths K (1976) Plasma steroid and protein hormone concentrations in patients with prostatic carcinoma before and during oestrogen therapy. Acta Endocrinol 81: 409–426
Hirst AE Jr, Bergman RT (1954) Carcinoma of the prostate in men 80 or more years old. Cancer 7: 136–141
Huggins C, Clark PJ (1940) Quantitative studies of prostatic secretion. II. The effect of castration and of estrogen injection on the normal and on the hyperplasia prostatic glands of dogs. J Exp Med 72: 747–458
Huggins C, Hodges CV (1941) Studies on prostatic cancer. I. The effect of castration, of estrogen and of androgen injection on serum phosphatases in metastatic carcinoma of the prostate. Cancer Res 1: 293–297
Huggins C, Stevens RE Jr, Hodges CV (1941) Studies on prostatic cancer. II. The effects of castration on advanced carcinoma of the prostate gland. Arch Surg 43: 209–223
King H, Diamond E, Lilienfeld AM (1963) Some epidemiological aspects of the prostate. J Chronic Dis 16: 117–153
Kley HK, Nieschlag E, Bidlingmaier F, Kruskemper HL (1974) Possible age-dependent influence of estrogens on the binding of testosterone in plasma of adult men. Horm Metab Res 6: 213–219
Kley HK, Nieschlag E, Krüskemper HL (1975) Age dependency of plasma oestrogen response to HCG and ACTH in man. Acta Endocrinol (Kbh) 79: 95–101
Lipton A, Sheemena L, Motel R, Harvey HA (1976) Urinary polyamine levels in patients with localized malignancy. Cancer 38: 1344–1347
Longcope C, Kato T, Horton R (1969) Conversion of blood androgens to estrogens in normal adult men and women. J Clin Invest 48: 2191–2201

Longcope C, Widrich W, Sawin CT (1972) The secretion of estrone and estradiol-17β by human testis. Steroids 20: 439–445

MacDonald PC, Grodin JM, Siiteri PK (1972) Dynamics of androgen and oestrogen secretion. In: Baird DT, Strong JA (eds) Control of gonadal steroid secretion. Williams & Wilkins, Baltimore, p 157

MacMahon B, Cole P, Lin TM, Lowe CR, Mirra AP, Ravnihar B, Salber EJ, Valaoras VG, Yuasa S (1970) Age at first birth and breast cancer risk. Bull WHO 43: 209–218

McGuire WL, Carbone PP, Sears ME, Escher GC (1975) Estrogen receptors in human breast cancers: an overview. In: McGuire WL, Carbone PP, Vollmer EP (eds) Estrogen receptors in human Breast cancer. Raven Press, New York, pp 1–7

McNeal JE (1970) Age-related changes in prostatic epithelium associated with carcinoma. In: Griffiths K, Pierrepoint CG (eds) Some aspects of the aetiology and biochemistry of prostatic cancer. Third Tenovus Workshop. Alpha Omega Alpha, Cardiff, pp 23–32

McNeal JE (1972) The prostate and prostatic urethra, a morphologic synthesis. J Urol 107: 1008–1016

McNeal JE (1975) Structure and pathology of the prostate. In: Goland M (ed) Normal and abnormal growth of the prostate. Thomas, Springfield, pp 55–68

Marton LJ, Russell DH, Levy CC (1973) Measurement of putrescine, spermidine and spermine in physiological fluids by use of amino acid analyser. Clin Chem 19: 923–926

Mobbs BG, Johnson IE, Connolly JG, Clark AF (1978) Androgen receptor assay in human benign and malignant prostatic tumour cytosol using protamine sulphate precipitation. J Steroid Biochem 9: 289–299

Pike A, Peeling WB, Harper ME, Pierrepoint CG, Griffiths K (1970) Testosterone metabolism in vivo by human prostatic tissue. Biochem J 120: 443–449

Pirke KM, Doerr P (1973) Age-related changes and interrelationship between plasma testosterone, oestradiol and testosterone-binding globulin in normal adult males. Acta Endocrinol (Kbh) 74: 792–807

Romas NA, Rose NR, Tannenbaum M (1979) Acid phosphatase: new developments. Hum Pathol 10: 501–512

Rosenblum MG, Durie BGM, Salmon SE, Russell DH (1978) Metabolism of [^{14}C]spermidine and [^{14}C]putrescine in normal volunteers and in cancer patients. Cancer Res 38: 3161–3163

Rokin ID (1977) Studies in the epidemiology of prostatic cancer: expanded sampling. Cancer Treat Rep 61: 173–180

Russell DH (1978) Polyamines as markers of tumour kinetics. In: Griffiths K, Pierrepont CG, Neville AM (eds) Tumour markers: determination and clinical role. Alpha Omega Alpha, Cardiff, pp 68–79

Sanford EJ, Drago JR, Rohner TJ, Kessler GF, Sheeman L, Lipton A (1975) Preliminary evaluation of urinary polyamines in the diagnosis of genito-urinary tract malignancy. J Urol 113: 218–221

Shain SA, Boesel RW (1978) Human prostate steroid hormone receptor quantitation. Invest Urol 16: 169–174

Snyder SH, Russell DH (1970) Polyamine synthesis in rapidly growing tissues. Fed Proc 29: 1575–1576

Steele R, Lees REM, Kraus AS, Rao C (1971) Sexual factors in the epidemiology of cancer of the prostate. J Chronic Dis 24: 29–37

Turkes A, Turkes AO, Joyce BG, Read GF, Riad-Fahmy D (1979) A sensitive solid phase enzyme-immunoassay for testosterone in plasma and saliva. Steroids 33: 347–351

Varkarakis M, Castro JE, Azzopardi JG (1970) Prognosis of stage 1 carcinoma of the prostate. Proc R Soc Med 63: 91

Vermeulen A, Stoica T, Verdonck L (1971) The apparent free testosterone concentration, an index of androgenicity. J Clin Endocrinol 33: 759–761

Vermeulen A, Rubens R, Verdonck L (1972) Testosterone secretion and metabolism in male senescence. J Clin Endocrinol 34: 730–735

Vihko P, Sajanti E, Janne O, Peltonen L, Vihko R (1978) Serum prostate-specific acid phosphatases: development and validation of a specific radioimmunoassay. Clin Chem 24: 1915–1923

Wallace DM, Chisholm GD, Hendry WF (1975) TNM classification for urological tumours (UICC). Br J Urol 47: 1–12

Walker RF, Read GF, Riad-Fahmy D (1978a) The radioimmunoassay of biologically active compounds in parotid fluid and plasma. In: Radioimmunoassay and related procedures in medicine, vol II. International Atomic Energy Agency, Vienna p 309

Walker RF, Riad-Fahmy D, Read GF (1978b) Adrenal status assessed by direct radioimmunoassay of cortisol in whole saliva and parotid saliva. Clin Chem 24: 1460–1463

Walker RF, Read GF, Riad-Fahmy D (1979) Radioimmunoassay of progesterone in saliva: application to the assessment of ovarian function. Clin Chem 25: 2030–2034

Walker RF, Wilson DW, Read GF, Riad-Fahmy D (1980) Assessment of testicular function by the radioimmunoassay of testosterone in saliva. Int J Andrology 3: 105–109

Williams-Ashman HG, Janne J, Coppoc GL, Geroch ME, Schenone A (1972a) New aspects of polyamine biosynthesis in eukaryotic organisms. Adv Enzyme Regul 10: 225

Williams-Ashman HG, Coppoc GL, Weber G (1972b) Imbalance in ornithine metabolism in hepatomas of different growth rates as expressed in formation of putrescine, spermidine and spermine. Cancer Res 32: 1924–1932

Williams-Ashman HG, Corti A, Sheth AR (1975) Formation and functions of aliphatic polyamines in the prostate gland and its secretions. In: Goland M (ed) Normal and abnormal growth of the prostate. Thomas, Springfield, p 222

Wynder EL, Mabuchi K, Whitmore WF (1971) Epidemiology of cancer of the prostate. Cancer 28: 344–360

Yam LT (1974) Clinical significance of the human acid phosphatases. A review. Am J Med 56: 604–616

Pathology and Natural History

R. C. B. Pugh

Department of Pathology, Institute of Urology, GB – London

1 Introduction

Prostatic carcinoma is by no means a homogeneous histopathological entity, and though more than 90% of the tumours arise from the acini there are less common forms, such as the ductal tumours, and a few much rarer types, including mucinous and carcinoid tumours, which are important because they can be difficult to diagnose and treat. Infiltration of the prostate by a urothelial carcinoma may cause similar problems.

2 Acinar Carcinoma

The acinar carcinoma arises in the peripheral and posterior parts of the gland, and in the fixed specimen may be noted to have a homogeneous solid, slightly granular cut surface, contrasting with the looser reticulated appearance that characterises the benign hyperplastic gland. Sometimes it is quite impossible to identify the malignant areas in fixed tissues, and much the best indication of tumour formation is the consistency of the unfixed tissue, which might have proved difficult to enucleate or cuts with increased resistance transurethrally. It is of immense help to the pathologist if any such areas in a surgical specimen are identified in some way so that they can receive particular attention in the laboratory. Poorly differentiated tumours are sometimes soft and yellowish in colour.

Microscopically the well-differentiated tumour is an adenocarcinoma consisting of small acini with a smooth inner lining and a single layer of regular cuboidal or low columnar cells. Their cytoplasm is pale and often finely granular, and the nuclei have a regular round or oval shape and are vesicular in type. Mitotic figures are extremely rare or entirely absent. In contrast, the benign hyperplastic acini are very much larger and have a crenated inner lining with papillary infoldings and a double layer of cells. Internally these are tall and columnar and radially arranged with pale cytoplasm and round regular, often quite darkly staining, nuclei; and externally there is a tangential layer of spindle-shaped cells with large pale vesicular nuclei (Fig. 1). A cribriform pattern of growth may be seen in both the benign hyperplastic and neoplastic glands (Fig. 2). The distinction between the single layer of cells in the malignant acini and the double layer in the benign hyperplastic ones is of crucial diagnostic importance, but it

Recent Results in Cancer Research, Vol. 78
© Springer-Verlag Berlin · Heidelberg 1981

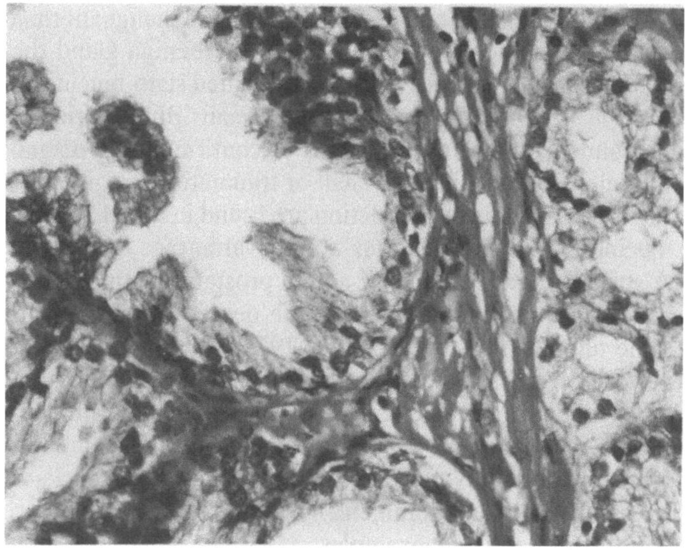

Fig. 1. Benign hyperplastic (*left*) and carcinomatous acini (*right*). H and E, 100× Enl × 5

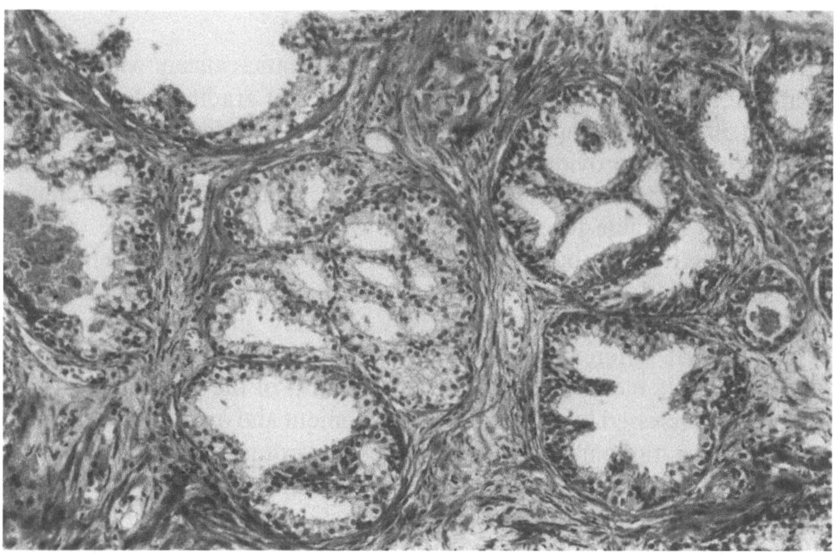

Fig. 2. Cribriform hyperplasia. H and E, 40× Enl × 5

should be remembered that benign atrophic acini are also usually lined by a single layer, though the acini tend to be rather large and of irregular size. Invasion of the seminal vesicles is diagnostic of tumour and of serious prognostic significance (Byar et al. 1972). Infiltration of perineural spaces is also diagnostic, but has no significance for overall prognosis (Pennington et al. 1967; Rodin et al. 1967). Striped muscle fibres are to be found in the fibromuscular stroma near the apex of the normal prostate, and care must be taken not to interpret close proximity of this muscle and acinar structures as evidence of tumour invasion (Kost and Ewan 1964). Mucus secretion is sometimes seen in the prostate and is commoner in the malignant than in the benign gland, but is not pathognomonic of neoplasia. In the benign gland the mucus is a neutral mucin whereas malignant cells secrete a sulphated sialo-mucin (Franks et al. 1964; Hukill and Vidone 1967). Staining by the Alcian Blue Periodic Acid-Schiff technique is recommended as a useful means of confirming the diagnosis of a well-differentiated tumour, especially in very small or traumatised fragments (Ansell 1976; Taylor 1979). Focal areas of mucin production are found in about 10% of prostatic carcinomas and a mucinous tumour occurs as a rare variant.

A striking feature of most if not all prostatic carcinomas is a considerable variation in histological appearances and in the degree of tumour differentiation in parts of the same tumour (Mostofi and Price 1973). With increasing de-differentiation the acinar pattern becomes less regular and is eventually lost altogether, to be replaced by sheets or slender trabeculae of cells. The cell morphology also changes and the cubico-columnar cells with their regular nuclei become replaced by pleomorphic cells whose cytoplasm is more eosinophilic and whose nuclei are large and vesicular and frequently contain prominent nucleoli. Mitotic figures are occasionally seen in the poorly differentiated examples.

2.1 Histological Grading

There have been many attempts to grade prostatic cancers with a view to assessing their malignant potential, but the very number of grading schemes published during the past 50 years (for full list of references see Mostofi 1976) points to the failure of many of them to provide a method that is simple and reproducible and capable of producing significant prognostic information. Many authors commend a particular scheme and are able to correlate grade with survival, incidence of metastases, and extent of the tumour, but many others are equally sceptical. Their views are perhaps best summarised by Willis (1948), who states that attempts at precise histological grading of malignant tumours are very arbitrary and unscientific, so that it is not surprising that different graders reach different conclusions on the same material. Broder's simple method forms the basis of most of the published classifications, and tumours are assessed by their acinar development and on the cell morphology. Mostofi (1976) divides tumours into three grades according to their differentiation (or the amount of glandular structure present) and anaplasia (which indicates the degree of aberration of cell morphology) (Figs. 3–5). Gleason (1966, 1977) and Gleason et al. (1974) have adopted a different approach, and evaluate the acinar pattern only. The primary and secondary patterns (found, respectively, in more than 50% and in the remainder of the acini) are given a numerical score and this 'pattern score' can be correlated with tumour stage and overall survival figures. Notwithstanding the misgivings of many graders there is good evidence that in general, the prognosis is better with well-differentiated than with poorly differentiated tumours (Kern 1978) and that there is a high incidence of lymph node metastases in patients with high-grade tumours, as is shown in a small unpublished series of cases studied in the St. Peter's Hospitals (O'Donoghue and Cameron, unpublished work; Table 1). In any series of specimens there is little practical difficulty in distinguishing the well-differentiated tumour (grade 1) from the very poorly differentiated one (grade 3), but discrepancies

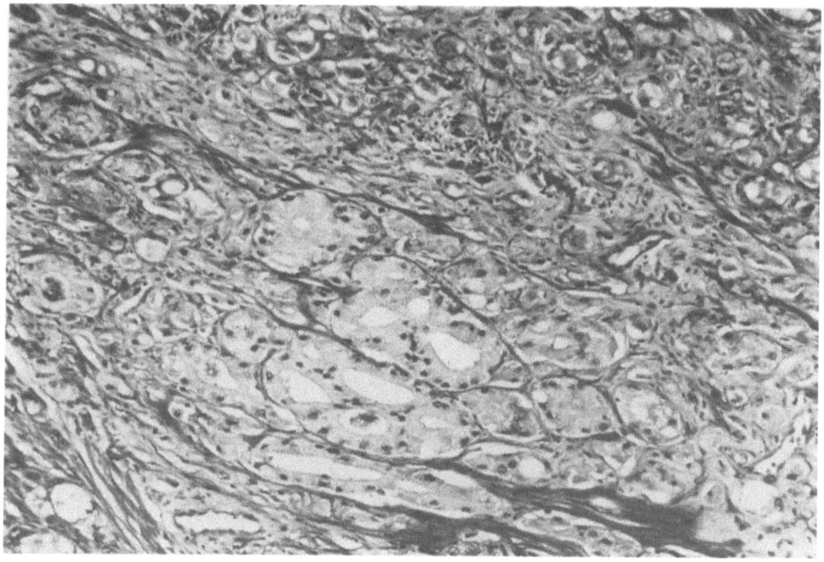

Fig. 3. Grade 1 carcinoma. Note small acini lined by regular cells in the lower half of the field. H and E, 40× Enl × 5

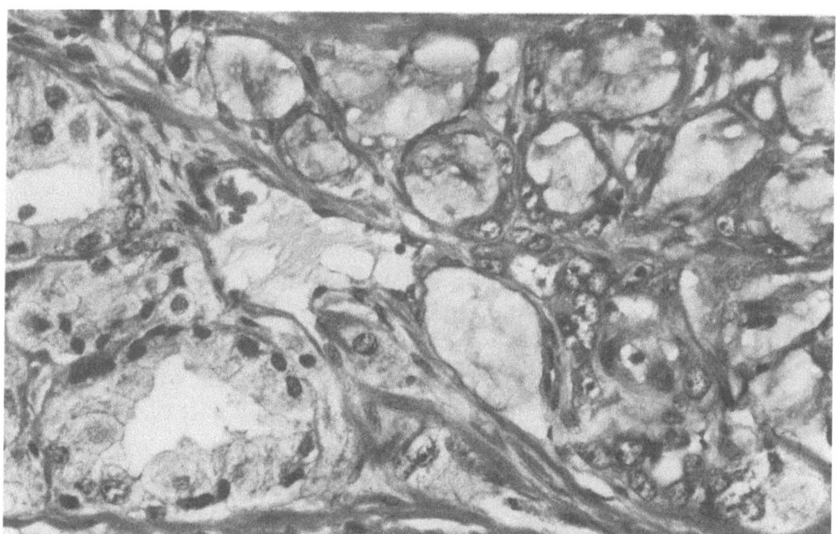

Fig. 4. Grade 2 carcinoma. There is some preservation of the acinar pattern but many nuclei are enlarged with very prominent nucleoli. The acini in the upper half of the field contain mucin. H and E, 100× Enl × 5

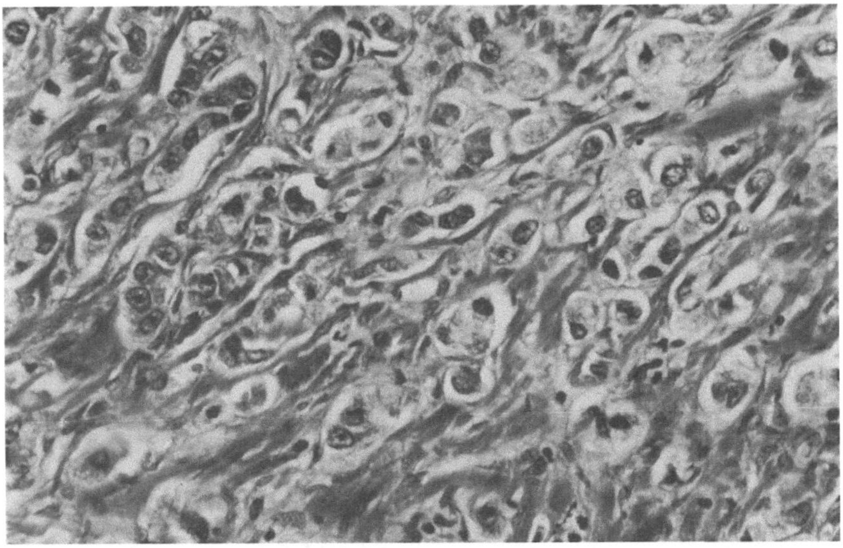

Fig. 5. Grade 3 carcinoma. No trace of an acinar pattern remains and the cells are arranged in columns. The nuclei are large and vesicular, with prominent nucleoli. H and E, 100× Enl × 5 (Figs. 3–5 were photographed from the same TUR specimen)

occur in the intervening grey area, i.e., with the grade 2 tumours, and clinicians must be aware of the practical difficulties as well as the limitations of tumour grading.

2.2 *Incidental Carcinoma*

Clinically, carcinoma of the prostate can be divided conveniently into three varieties – incidental, clinically manifest and occult. The incidental tumour, the TO pT1 tumour of the UICC system of classification (Wallace et al. 1975), has been and still is the subject of speculation regarding the criteria for its diagnosis and the best method of treatment, if indeed any treatment is required at all. Histological diagnosis is usually not difficult if the lesion is small, well-circumscribed, and well-differentiated (Fig. 6), but the possibility that a small malignant area is only part of a much more extensive

Table 1. Correlation of grade of primary tumour and incidence of histologically proved regional lymph node metastases (29 cases). O'Donoghue and Cameron (unpublished work)

Grade of prostatic primary	Tumour in nodes	
	Absent	Present
1	16	1
2	2	4
3	0	6

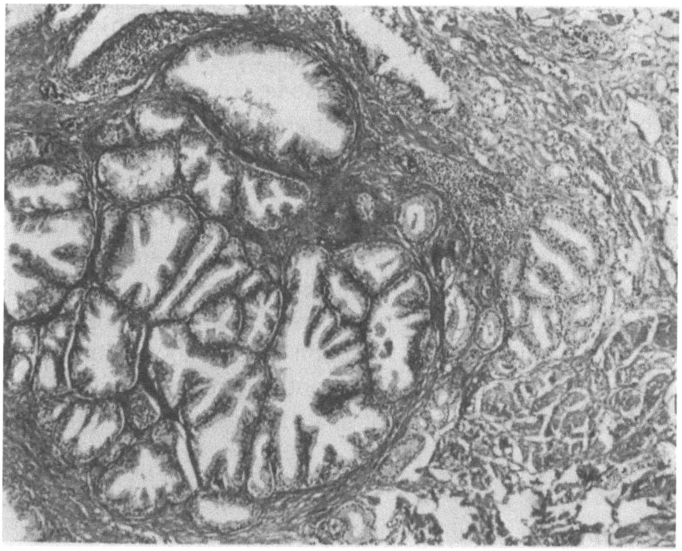

Fig. 6. Incidental (focal) carcinoma. The tumour is well circumscribed and well differentiated. H and E, 16× Enl × 5

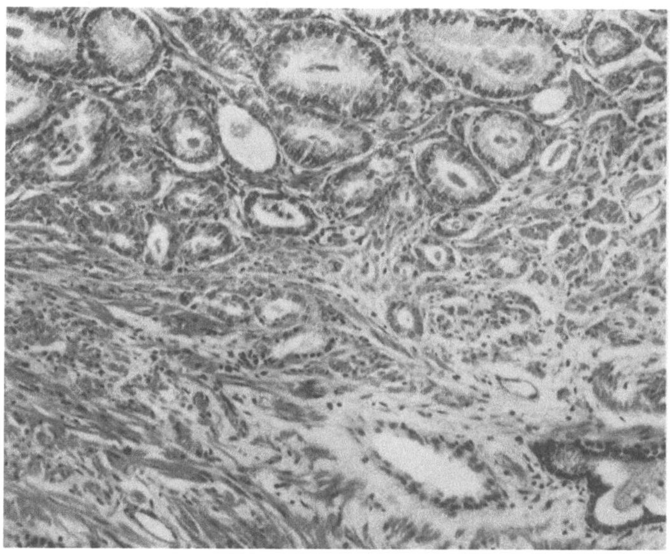

Fig. 7. Infiltration of fibromuscular stroma at the margin of a small focus of carcinoma. H and E, 40× Enl × 5

tumour should be suspected immediately when the margins are ragged and there is peripheral infiltration (Fig. 7). Small areas of 'focal' carcinoma are known to occur in up to 20% of apparently benign glands, and their numbers increase with advancing age of the patient and increasing amount of the gland sampled (Whitmore 1956). The clinical significance of these foci is debatable. Greene and Simon (1955) noted that about 10% of their patients found to have them died of cancer and that a low-grade tumour and small size were favourable prognostic features. Other authors have reached similar conclusions (Barnes et al. 1976), and Jewett (1975) suggested a subdivision into two groups – stages A1 (focal) and A2 (diffuse) – indicating in addition that the grade should also be recorded. He recommended that the A1 lesions, which are usually well-differentiated, be left alone without treatment and remarked that the A2 tumour, when of high grade, usually progresses and requires treatment. Golimbu et al. (1978) reviewed a series of 53 patients with clinical stage A1, A2, B1, and B2 tumours and found that one-third of the unsuspected tumours were stage A2, with a higher incidence of poor differentiation and lymph node metastases than in their A1 and B1 cases. Even when the problems of grading can be overcome satisfactorily the difficulty of assessing tumor size remains, and probably the best the pathologist can do with a transurethral resection (TUR) specimen is to record the number of the fragments of tissue in it which contain tumour. Differential sampling of the gland may also be of help in arriving at a true assessment (O'Donoghue and Pugh 1977).

2.3 Clinically Manifest Carcinoma

About one-third to a half of the patients who have clinically manifest carcinoma (UICC stages T1–T4) have distant metastases when they are first seen (O'Donoghue et al. 1976). Microscopically the tumour is an adenocarcinoma (grades 1–3), and in the less well-differentiated types slender trabeculae of cells arranged 'in Indian file' are seen invading the stroma (Fig. 8). Invasion of the prostatic capsule is indicative of an aggressive tumour, and invasion of the seminal vesicles may presage lymph node involvement in more than 80% of cases (Arduino and Glucksman 1962). Lymphatic invasion occurs with high-grade tumours, and in the series of cases reported in the

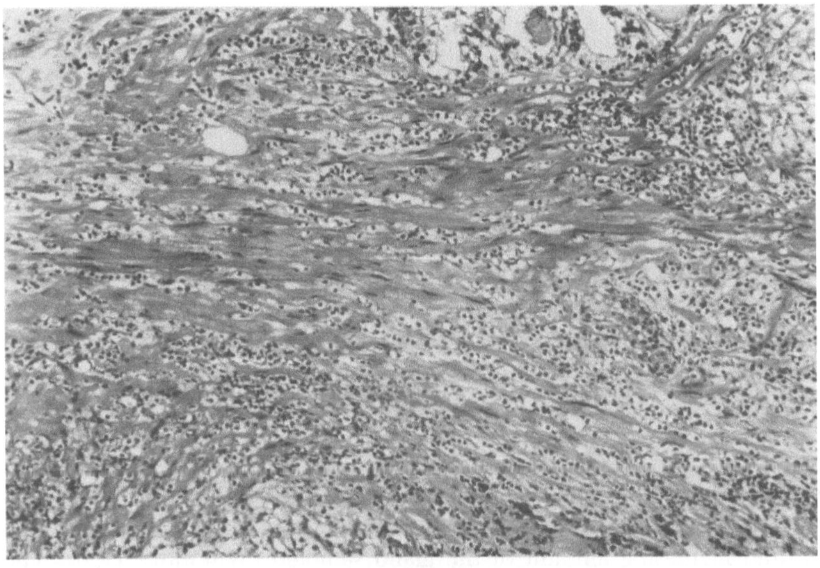

Fig. 8. Stromal invasion by slender trabeculae of tumour cells (Indian file infiltration). Lymphocytic infiltration may mimic this lesion. H and E, 40× Enl ×5

literature reviewed by O'Donoghue et al. (1976), regional nodal metastases were present in about 20% of T1 and T2 cases and in 50% of T3 cases. Bones of the pelvis and sacrum, lumbar spine, femora, thoracic spine, and ribs may contain metastases, which are usually osteosclerotic. Terminally there is haematogenous spread to the viscera, the lungs, liver, and kidney being the organs most affected. The precise identification of tumours at the bladder base may be a problem for both the cystoscopist, who needs to know whether there is a carcinoma of the bladder or of the prostate to treat, and the histopathologist. Microscopically any hint of an acinar pattern would immediately suggest a prostatic carcinoma, but in its absence the finding of prominent nucleoli and cells in an Indian file pattern of infiltration would favour a prostatic tumour, whereas a squamous tendency and an abundance of mitoses would be more suggestive of a bladder tumour. Additional help may come from the localisation of acid phosphatase in the cells by an immunohistological method which can be applied to formalin-fixed paraffin embedded material (Jöbsis et al. 1978). Benign and neoplastic cells will both stain, and a disadvantage of the method is that as a tumour becomes less well-differentiated so the staining becomes less intense. The prognosis of prostatic cancer depends on its grade and the extent of local spread to the vesicles and other adjacent tissues and also (but not for discussion here) on its stage, the presence of lymph node and distant metastases, and the treatment that is given.

2.4 Occult Carcinoma

The patient with the occult form of the disease, sometimes known as silent metastasising carcinoma, presents with metastatic disease and after investigation is found to have a hitherto unsuspected primary in the prostate. From the pathological point of view the appearances are in no way different from those in the clinically manifest form. The immunohistochemical method of localising acid phosphatase may assist in the diagnosis.

3 Biopsy Techniques

Diagnostic biopsy with the use of Tru-Cut needles through the perineum or rectum or Franzén needles transrectally gives reliable results (Williams et al. 1967; Prout 1973) and is usually free of serious complications, though seeding of cancer cells has been recorded (Addonizio and Kapoor 1976). The fine-needle biopsy (Franzén et al. 1960) has the distinct advantage that it can be carried out as an out-patient procedure in an unanaesthetised patient and provides a cytological diagnosis (Fig. 9), whereas a tissue diagnosis is possible with the larger needles (Fig. 10) (Hendry and Williams 1971). Some workers have been able to assess the grade of a tumour (Esposti 1971) as well as its response to treatment in material obtained with the Franzén and larger needles (Ziegler et al. 1974). Squamous metaplasia of duct epithelium in transurethral resection specimens is a good indication that the patient has been taking oestrogens, and cytoplasmic vacuolation and some degree of nuclear pyknosis in the tumour cells are indicative of response to treatment (Fig. 11).

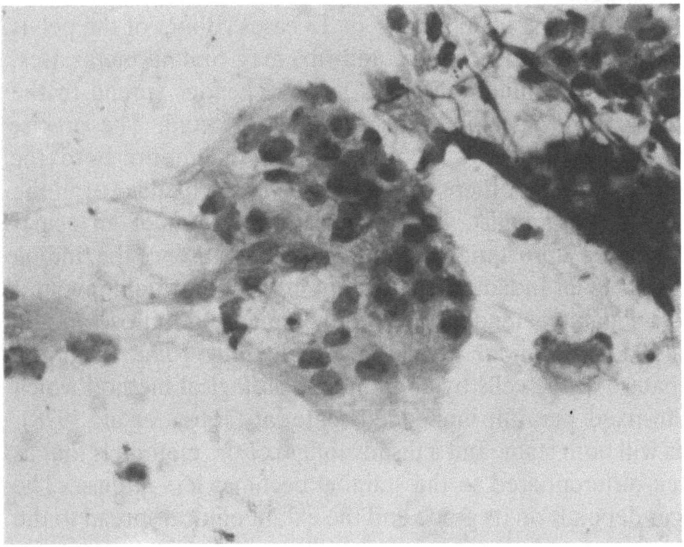

Fig. 9. Franzén needle aspirate. Note the large nuclei (with prominent nucleoli) and indistinct cell outlines in the central clump of carcinoma cells. H and E, 100× Enl × 5

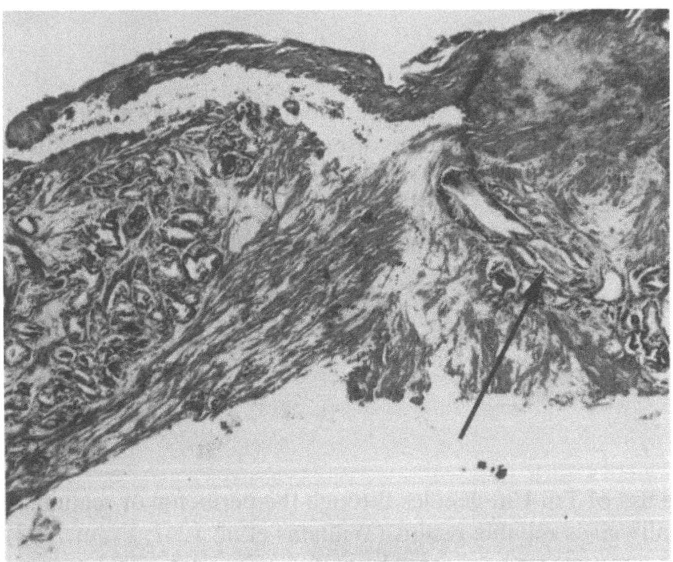

Fig. 10. Tru-Cut needle biopsy of prostate. Note the crowded carcinomatous acini (*left*) and the infiltration of perineural spaces (*right*). H and E, 16× Enl × 5

The differential diagnosis of tumours at the bladder base has already been referred to. Carcinoma of the rectum may be suspected in a patient with a pelvic mass, but the presence of nucleoli in the prostatic tumour and their relative rarity in rectal tumours may help to distinguish the two in biopsy material. An important clinical differential diagnosis is granulomatous prostatitis, which often produces a hard gland, but biopsy should provide the correct diagnosis.

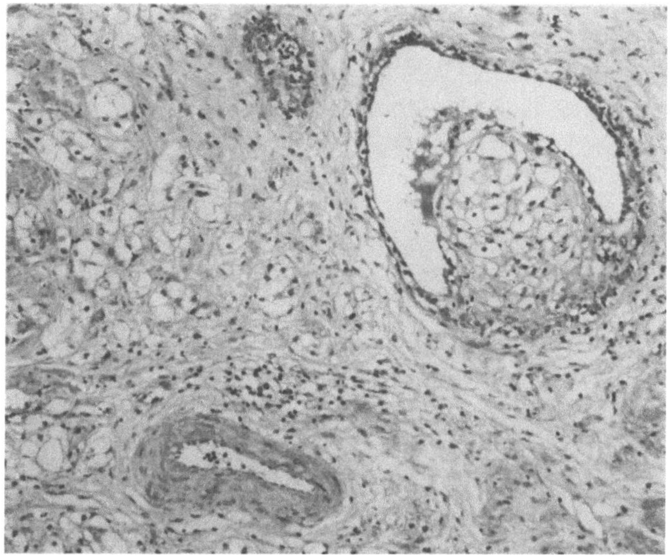

Fig. 11. Oestrogen-treated carcinoma. Note the signet ring squamous metaplasia of duct epithelium and the cytoplasmic vacuolation and nuclear pyknosis of the tumour cells which are invading the stroma. H and E, 40× Enl × 5

4 Carcinoma of the Prostatic Ducts

The tumours arising in the prostatic ducts are an interesting group, which differ in structure and behaviour from the very much commoner acinar type (Kopelson et al. 1978). The ducts dip into the stroma of the gland from the prostatic urethra and are lined at their mouths by transitional epithelium continuous with the urethral epithelium, and in their deeper parts by cubico-columnar cells. The ductal system may be involved when there is a transitional cell carcinoma of the bladder or urethra, the tumour either growing down the duct lumen or occurring as an in situ change in the lining cells. A bladder tumour which invades the prostate is classified as a stage T4a or pT4a tumour in the UICC system, but it is important to appreciate that the tumour which remains within the duct has a very much better prognosis than the one which subsequently transgresses the basement membrane and invades the fibromuscular stroma. For this reason it has been suggested that it would be worthwhile subdividing the group into two: stage 4aa indicating intraduct tumour, and 4ab denoting interstitial involvement (Pugh, to be published). Occasionally a transitional cell carcinoma of the ducts arises without a preceding or concomitant urothelial tumour elsewhere (Karpas and Mourigis 1969) or may accompany an adenocarcinoma in the prostate (Ende et al. 1963). Rhamy et al. (1973) reported some such cases and noted that they occurred in patients who were younger than the majority of prostatic tumour patients; the serum acid phosphatase was not raised and the tumours responded poorly to hormones and radiotherapy.

Tumours arising in the primary ducts, that is, those parts of the ductal system in close relation to the urethra, are columnar-celled papillary tumours (Fig. 12), and the

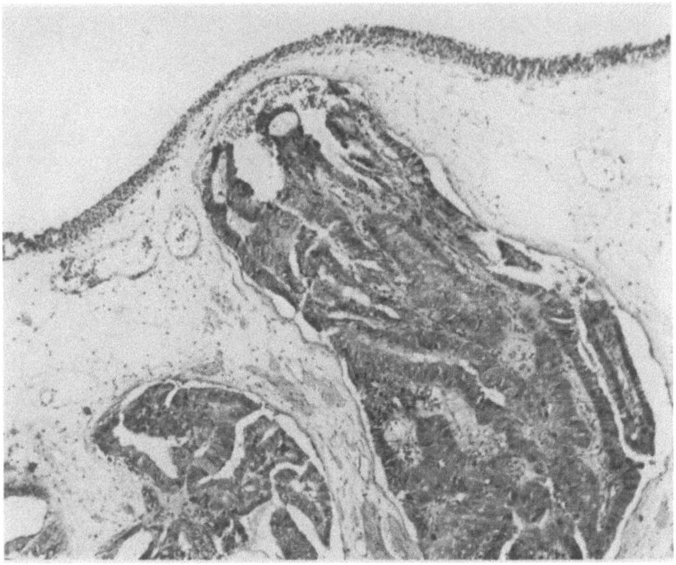

Fig. 12. Columnar-celled papillary carcinoma of the primary ducts distending the duct lumen. H and E, 16× Enl × 5

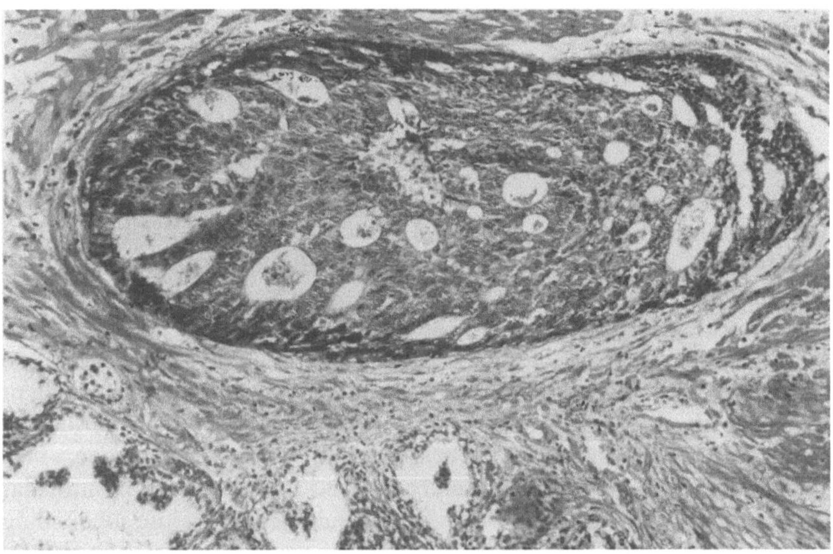

Fig. 13. Cribriform carcinoma of the secondary ducts. Note the benign hyperplastic acini in the lower part of the field. H and E, 40× Enl × 5

secondary, or deeper ducts, give origin to cribriform or comedo-type neoplasms (Fig. 13). Clinically there are no significant differences between either of these groups and the acinar tumours in respect of presentation, age of incidence, levels of serum acid phosphatase, or findings on rectal examination (Greene et al. 1979). But the survival rate figures are not encouraging and, in general, the secondary duct tumours are less

Table 2. Data on 262 cases of prostatic duct carcinoma

Type	Incidence	Histology	Spread		% 5-year survival rate
			Ducts	Stroma	
Primary duct	8 (0.19%)	Columnar cell papillary	↑↑ ↓	+	42.8
Secondary duct	47 (1.1%)	Cribriform comedo	↑ ↓↓	++	24.2
Mixed	207 (4.8%)	Primary or secondary plus acinar		+	45.6

From an analysis of 4,286 cases of prostatic carcinoma by Dube et al. (1973)

responsive to endocrine therapy and more malignant than the primary duct ones, as is well demonstrated in the series reported by Dube et al. (1973) (Table 2). It will be noted that duct tumours are rare, that mixed forms occur more often than single ones, and that in all types spread either within the duct system or into the stroma is likely.

5 Less Common Tumours

There is controversy regarding the very rare endometrioid carcinoma, so called because of its histological similarity to the uterine tumour. This was first described by Melicow and Tannenbaum (1971), who suggested that it might originate from the prostatic utricle. The serum acid phosphatase was not raised in their six cases and, because of the possibility of a Müllerian origin, oestrogen administration and orchidectomy were considered to be contraindicated. Subsequent reports of regression of such a tumour after orchidectomy (Young and Lagios 1973) and of ultrastructural findings (Zaloudek et al. 1975) have cast some doubts on Melicow's and Tannenbaum's beliefs regarding the precise site of initial tumour formation, and many believe that this is not so much a separate entity as a variant of primary duct carcinoma.

True mucinous carcinomas occasionally occur (Fig. 14) (Sika and Buckley 1964; Joshi et al. 1967) and are reported to be less invasive and less responsive to oestrogens than the acinar tumours.

The prostate may be invaded by a squamous carcinoma, in very much the same way as has been described for the transitional cell tumours (Fig. 15), and very occasionally a squamous carcinoma develops as a complication of prolonged oestrogen therapy. The squamous metaplasia which very commonly occurs in the surviving tissue immediately next to an area of infarction is not of sinister significance but needs to be distinguished from tumour.

Azzopardi and Evans (1971) reported a case of adenocarcinoma of the prostate in which there were areas with the features of a carcinoid tumour, and also found argentaffin cells in a significant number of other prostatic carcinomas (Figs. 16 and 17). Montasser et al. (1979) recorded a similar association of adenocarcinoma and

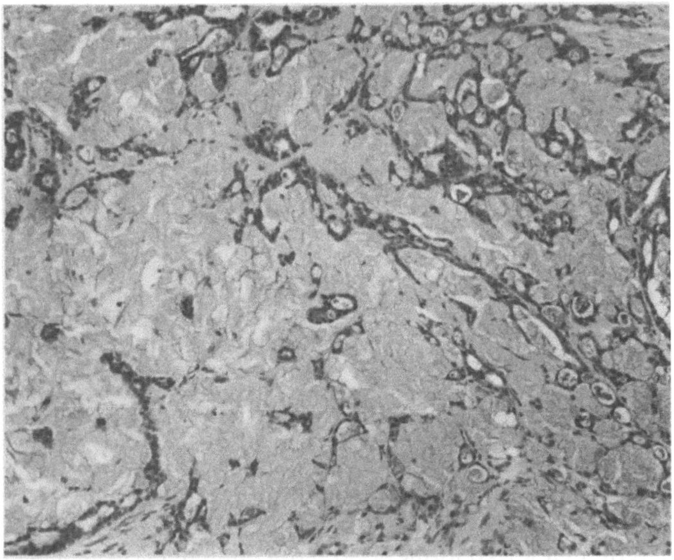

Fig. 14. Mucinous carcinoma. Alcian Blue-PAS, 40× Enl × 5

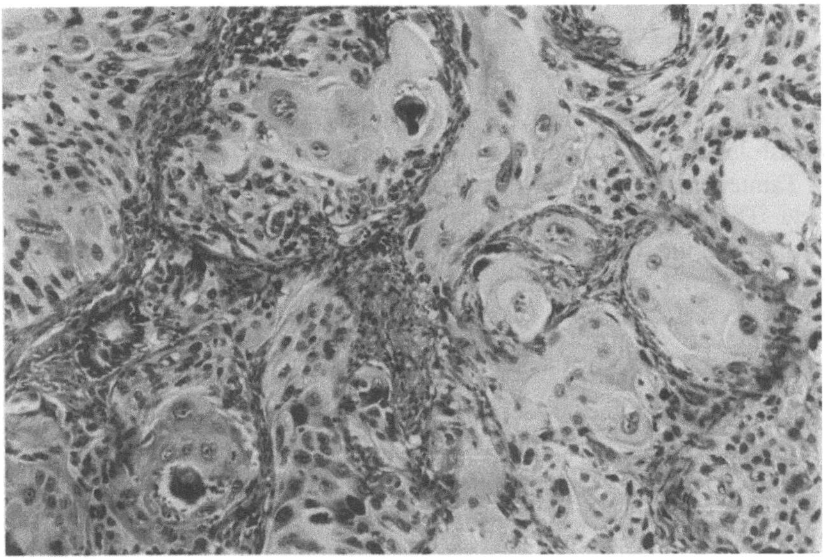

Fig. 15. Squamous carcinoma. H and E, 40× Enl × 5

carcinoid and Wasserstein and Goldman (1979) have described a case of pure primary prostatic carcinoid. The significance of the carcinoid elements in terms of prognosis is not yet known.

Single cases of adenoid cystic carcinoma (Kramer et al. 1978) and of a tumour interpreted as a primary yolk-sac tumour of the prostate (Benson et al. 1978) have also been described.

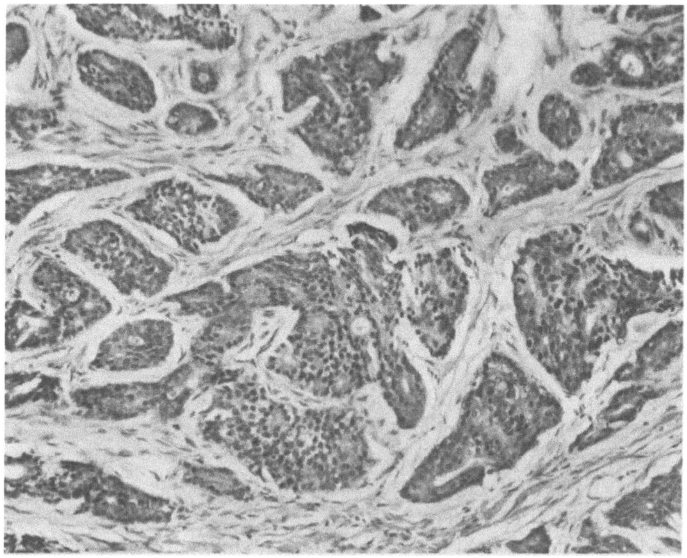

Fig. 16. Carcinoid tumour. H and E, 40× Enl × 5

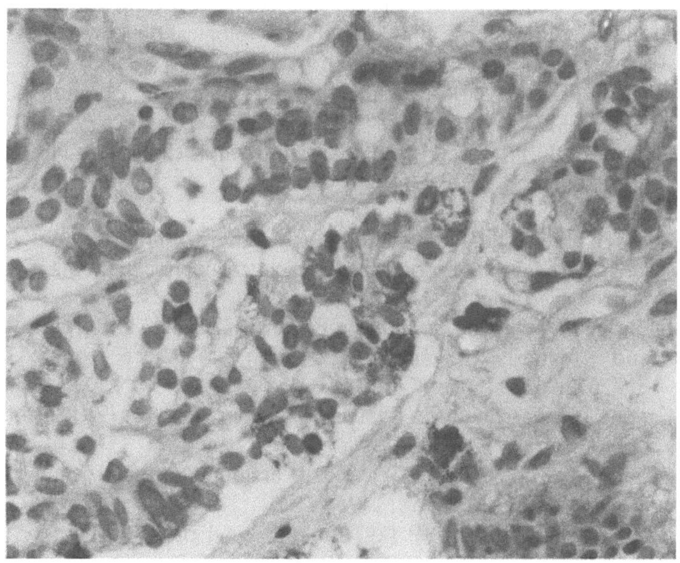

Fig. 17. Carcinoid tumour. Intracytoplasmic argentaffin granules. Diazo, 160× Enl × 5

The histological diagnosis of prostatic carcinoma may be relatively straightforward and simple. The real problems lie with the apparently small focus of tumour and with the efforts that are needed to estimate its true extent – that is, whether it is an A1 or an A2 lesion. Grading is never easy but should always be attempted, as it may give the clinician useful prognostic information.

6 References

Addonizio JC, Kapoor SN (1976) Perineal seeding of prostatic cancer after needle biopsy. Urology 8: 513–515

Ansell ID (1976) The prostate: histopathology. In: Innes Williams D, Chisholm GD (eds) Scientific foundations of urology, vol II. Heinemann, London, p 334

Arduino LJ, Glucksman MA (1962) Lymph node metastases in early carcinoma of the prostate. J Urol 88: 91–93

Azzopardi JG, Evans DJ (1971) Argentaffin cells in prostatic carcinoma; differentiation from lipofuscin and melanin in prostatic epithelium. J Pathol Bacteriol 104: 247–251

Barnes R, Hirst A, Rosenquist R (1976) Early carcinoma of the prostate: Comparison of stages A and B. J Urol 115: 404–405

Benson RC, Segura JW, Carney JA (1978) Primary yolk-sac (endodermal sinus) tumor of the prostate. Cancer 41: 1395–1398

Byar DP, Mostofi FK, Veterans Cooperative Urological Research Group (1972) Carcinoma of the prostate – prognostic features in 208 radical prostatectomies. Cancer 30: 5–13

Dube VE, Farrow GM, Greene LF (1973) Prostatic adenocarcinoma of ductal origin. Cancer 32: 402–409

Ende N, Woods LP, Shelley HS (1963) Carcinoma originating in ducts surrounding the prostatic urethra. Am J Clin Pathol 40: 183–189

Esposti PL (1971) Cytologic malignancy grading of prostatic carcinoma by transrectal aspiration biopsy. Scand J Urol Nephrol 5: 199–209

Franks LM, O'Shea JD, Thompson AER (1964) Mucin in the prostate: a histochemical study in normal glands, latent, clinical and colloid cancers. Cancer 17: 983–991

Franzén S, Giertz G, Zajicek J (1960) Cytological diagnosis of prostatic tumours by transrectal aspiration biopsy. A preliminary report. Br J Urol 32: 193–196

Gleason DF (1966) Classification of prostatic carcinomas. Cancer Chemother Rep 50: 125–128

Gleason DF (1977) Histologic grading and clinical staging of prostatic carcinoma. In: Tannenbaum M (ed) Urologic pathology – the prostate. Lee and Febiger, Philadelphia, pp 171–197

Gleason DF, Mellinger GT, Veterans Administration Cooperative Urological Research Group (1974) Prediction of prognosis for prostatic adenocarcinoma by combined histological grading and clinical staging. J Urol 111: 58–64

Golimbu M, Schinella R, Morales P, Kurusu S (1978) Differences in pathological characteristics and prognosis of clinical A2 prostatic cancer from A1 and B disease. J Urol 119: 618–622

Greene LF, Farrow GM, Ravits JM, Tomera FM (1979) Prostatic adenocarcinoma of ductal origin. J Urol 121: 303–305

Greene LF, Simon HB (1955) Occult carcinoma of the prostate: Clinical and therapeutic study of 83 cases. JAMA 158: 1494–1498

Hendry WF, Williams JP (1971) Transrectal prostatic biopsy. Br Med J 4: 595–597

Hukill PB, Vidone RA (1967) Histochemistry of mucus and other polysaccharides in tumours. II. Carcinoma of prostate. Lab Invest 16: 395–406

Jewett H (1975) Present status of radical prostatectomy for Stages A and B prostatic cancer. Urol Clin North Am 2: 105–124

Jöbsis AC, De Vries GP, Anholt RRH, Sanders GTB (1978) Demonstration of the prostatic origin of metastases. Cancer 41: 1788–1793

Joshi DP, Seery WH, Neier CR (1967) Mucogenic adenocarcinoma of the prostate. J Urol 98: 241–243

Karpas CM, Mourigis B (1969) Primary transitional cell carcinoma of prostate gland: possible pathogenesis and relationship to reserve cell hyperplasia of prostatic periurethral ducts. J Urol 101: 201–205

Kern WH (1978) Well-differentiated adenocarcinoma of the prostate. Cancer 41: 2046–2054
Kopelson G, Harisiadis L, Romas NA, Veenema RJ, Tannenbaum M (1978) Periurethral prostatic duct carcinoma. Cancer 42: 2894–2902
Kost LV, Ewan GW (1964) Occurrence and significance of striated muscle within the prostate. J Urol 92: 703–704
Kramer SA, Bredael JJ, Krueger RP (1978) Adenoid cystic carcinoma of the prostate: report of a case. J Urol 120: 383–384
Melicow MM, Tannenbaum M (1971) Endometrial carcinoma of uterus masculinus (prostatic utricle). Report of 6 cases. J Urol 106: 892–902
Montasser AY, Ong MG, Mehta VT (1979) Carcinoid tumour of the prostate associated with adenocarcinoma. Cancer 44: 307–310
Mostofi FK (1976) Problems of grading carcinoma of prostate. Semin Oncol 3: 161–169
Mostofi FK, Price EB (1973) Tumors of the male genital system: Atlas of tumor pathology, fasc. 8. AFIP, Washington DC, pp 196–258
O'Donoghue EPN, Pugh RCB (1977) Early diagnosis of prostatic carcinoma: the role of transurethral resection. Br J Urol 49: 705–710
O'Donoghue EPN, Shridhar P, Sherwood T, Williams JP, Chisholm GD (1976) Lymphography and pelvic lymphadenectomy in carcinoma of the prostate. Br J Urol 48: 689–696
Prout GRJ (1973) Proceedings: diagnosis and staging of prostatic cancer. Cancer 32: 1096–1103
Pennington JW, Prentiss RJ, Howe G (1967) Radical prostatectomy for cancer – significance of perineural lymphatic invasion. J Urol 97: 1075–1077
Pugh RCB (to be published) The diagnosis of carcinoma in situ of the urinary bladder. In: Hendry WF (ed) Recent advances in urology, no. 3. Churchill Livingstone, Edingburgh London New York
Rhamy RK, Buchanan RD, Spalding MJ (1973) Intraductal carcinoma of the prostate gland. J Urol 109: 457–460
Rodin AE, Larson DL, Roberts DK (1967) Nature of the perineural space invaded by prostatic carcinoma. Cancer 20: 1772–1779
Sika JV, Buckley JJ (1964) Mucus-forming adenocarcinoma of prostate. Cancer 17: 949–952
Taylor NS (1979) Histochemistry in the diagnosis of early prostatic carcinoma. Hum Pathol 10: 513–520
Wallace DM, Chisholm GD, Hendry WF (1975) TNM classification of urological tumours – UICC 1974. Br J Urol 47: 1–12
Wasserstein PW, Goldman RL (1979) Primary carcinoid of prostate. Urology 13: 318–320
Whitmore WF (1956) Hormone therapy in prostatic cancer. Am J Med 21: 697–713
Williams JP, Still BM, Pugh RCB (1967) The diagnosis of prostatic cancer: cytological and biochemical studies using the Franzén biopsy needle. Br J Urol 39: 549–554
Willis RA (1948) Pathology of tumours. Butterworths, London, p 21
Young BW, Lagios MD (1973) Endometrial (papillary) carcinoma of the prostatic utricle – response to orchiectomy. Cancer 32: 1293–1300
Zaloudek C, Williams JW, Kempson RL (1976) "Endometrial" adenocarcinoma of the prostate. Cancer 37: 2255–2262
Ziegler H, Völter D, Schubert GE (1974) Morphological criteria for the control of carcinoma of the prostate with estrogen therapy. Int Urol Nephrol 6: 195–200

Diagnostic Imaging

H. Mamtora, M. R. Gowland, and I. Isherwood

Department of Diagnostic Radiology, University of Manchester, GB – Manchester

1 Introduction

Despite the incidence of both benign and malignant prostatic disease and the significant morbidity and mortality resulting from it, prostatic imaging has played a minor role in clinical management. Assessment of patients has depended traditionally upon clinical methods and indirect imaging techniques including excretion urography and cysto-urethrography, with the occasional addition of more invasive methods. Diagnosis of cancer has relied mainly upon the discovery of a palpable abnormality by rectal examination and upon subsequent histological confirmation in tissue removed by biopsy, transurethral resection, or enucleation of an adenoma. The importance of early diagnosis of malignancy is emphasised by the observation that 10%–20% of men in their sixties and 20%–40% of those over 75 years have latent prostatic cancer (Blacklock 1977). Recognisable induration of the prostate is of limited value in early malignancy, being present in fewer than 25% of patients.

In all forms of prostatic disease reproducible evaluation of prostatic morphology is important. Impressions obtained from rectal examination alone are subjective and prone to error. In benign prostatic hyperplasia the efficacy of various new hormone preparations in influencing the hyperplastic process needs to be evaluated and the potential role of imaging techniques resides in accurate objective evaluation of gland size throughout a series of observations in a controlled clinical trial.

In the surgical treatment of prostatic hyperplasia controversy still exists, especially about how much gland resection is required to produce clinical improvement. In this respect it is useful to delineate the areas of resection to compare with the pre-operative appearances. Volume estimation is useful in deciding the correct surgical approach for patients with benign prostatic hyperplasia (BPH).

The introduction of ultrasound and computed tomography have enabled direct non-invasive imaging of the prostate. Whilst the precise role of these newer imaging methods has not yet been evaluated fully, initial studies have been very encouraging (Whittingham and Bishop 1973; Miller et al. 1973; Watanabe et al. 1971, 1975, 1977; Boyce et al. 1976; Harada et al. 1979, Resnick et al. 1977; Peeling et al. 1979; Sukov et al. 1977; Brizel et al. 1979).

In this review of prostatic imaging, attention will be focussed on the techniques of ultrasound and computed tomography with brief mention of other available methods (Table 1). The role of lymphography and isotope bone scanning in prostatic cancer is discussed in Chapters 7 and 8, respectively, and will not be considered further here.

Recent Results in Cancer Research, Vol. 78
© Springer-Verlag Berlin · Heidelberg 1981

Table 1. Techniques for prostatic imaging

Indirect	Direct
Plain film	Ultrasonography
Intravenous urography	Computed tomography
Simple cystography	Radionuclide scanning
Cystourethrography	Prostatography
Arteriography and venography	
Seminal vesiculography	

2 Indirect Radiological Techniques

2.1 Plain Film

The role of the plain film is limited to the detection of calculi or calcification within the prostatic area and of metastatic disease in the skeleton. Metastatic spread most commonly occurs to the lumbar spine and pelvis; lesions from prostatic cancer are predominantly of the sclerotic type and present either as discrete dense areas or an ill-defined diffuse reaction. The pattern of distribution of metastases is 80% sclerotic, 4% lytic, and 12% mixed (MacCallum and Colapinto 1970).

2.2 Intravenous Urography (IVU)

The IVU is commonly employed to provide information about the state of the upper urinary tract, and may demonstrate vesical abnormalities associated with bladder outlet obstruction. There may be no visible evidence of renal function on one or both sides, or alternatively, hydronephrotic changes may be evident.

Prostatic enlargement may cause indentation of the bladder base, which may also be elevated, but the latter finding only becomes significant when there is associated deformity of the lower ureters (Vermooten and Schweinsberg 1964). Changes described in the bladder include detrusor muscle hypertrophy, trabeculation, and formation of diverticula; residual urine may be demonstrated on both the preliminary and the postvoiding films. Abrams et al. (1968, 1979) studied 201 patients with prostatism by excretion urography and dynamic pressure/flow studies to assess the significance of these radiological signs. Both trabeculation and diverticula were found to be significantly related to bladder instability but not to bladder outlet obstruction.

Indentation of the bladder base was associated with outlet obstruction, and the larger the defect the greater was the incidence of associated obstruction. Bladder instability was noted in 56% of their patients. Upper urinary tract dilatation (unilateral or bilateral) was seen in only 5% and in none was subsequent management altered by this finding. Similar conclusions have been reached by Marshall et al. (1975) in a group of patients with acute retention of urine before prostatectomy.

Boerema (1972) questions the necessity of pre-operative excretion urography after analysing 125 examinations on patients with BPH. Of the urograms in this series, 85%

were normal, and whilst in the remainder a variety of abnormalities were demonstrated, including absence of visible function and hydronephrosis, in no case was any additional treatment necessary except in a small number with bladder calculi.

Residual urine may be seen on the postvoiding film, but this appears only in the decompensated phase of bladder outlet obstruction. In the compensated phase, the bladder may empty completely even in the presence of severe outlet obstruction.

Griffiths and Castro (1970) evaluated the accuracy of planimetric measurement of residual urine, and correlated its volume with clinical and radiographic findings. Though there was a close correlation between radiological postmicturition residue and its actual volume measured by catheterisation, there was no association between residual volume and thickness of bladder wall, trabeculation, length of prostatic urethra on cysto-urethrography, urine flow rate, or digital assessment of prostatic size.

While the precise role of excretion urography still needs to be defined, routine investigation of the urinary tract in this manner is likely to continue, to provide both information about the upper urinary tract and indirect evidence of prostatic disease and associated changes within the bladder.

2.3 Simple Cystography and Cysto-urethrography

Cystography and cysto-urethrography can be used for the assessment of bladder diverticula and filling defects and of changes in the prostatic urethra secondary to prostatic disease. Thumann (1951) described a method of calculating prostatic size on cysto-urethrography, but his technique is elaborate and carries a measurement error rate of about 20%.

The association between bladder instability and outlet obstruction has already been mentioned. A large number of patients have recently been investigated by pressure/flow studies before and after elective prostatectomy (Abrams et al. 1979). Many symptoms attributed to obstruction were found to be due to bladder instability, which was demonstrated in 60% of the patients; this incidence dropped to 25% postoperatively. The presence of instability in the absence of obstruction underlines the importance of urodynamic assessment in patients with frequency and urgency. It is also useful in patients who have had a prostatectomy, when persistent symptoms may be due to either instability or residual obstruction (Turner-Warwick et al. 1973).

2.4 Prostatic Venography and Arteriography

Contrast medium introduced into the prostatic venous plexus has been used to differentiate benign and malignant disease (Laubenberger and Berghaus 1966). Prostatic adenoma results in cranial and lateral displacement of the inferior vesical vein, which may be stretched and elongated. Obstruction and displacement of the veins forming the plexus have been described in prostatic carcinoma.

The prostate is supplied by the internal pudendal, inferior vesical, and middle haemorrhoidal arteries. Prostatic arteriography has been utilised to differentiate between BPH and cancer (Bobbio et al. 1959; Goerttler 1977; Belli et al. 1978). The normal prostatic angle formed by the inferior vesical and middle haemorrhoidal arteries is about 80°; elevation and displacement of the inferior vesical artery in BPH results in an increase of this angle. In carcinoma, enlargement and tortuosity of prostatic arteries, pathological vessels, tumour blush, arteriovenous shunting, and hypervascularity of the urethral branches have been described.

Goerttler (1977) performed bilateral selective arteriography in a group of 38 patients with prostatic disease. In 18 patients with the clinical diagnosis of BPH, arteriography revealed carcinoma. In ten patients with clinically suspected carcinoma, five were diagnosed malignant at arteriography.

The invasive nature of the procedure, necessity for bilateral catheterisation of femoral arteries, the inherent risks associated with contrast media and availability of newer, non-invasive imaging methods negate the potential value of this technique.

2.5 Seminal Vesiculography

Seminal vesiculograms may be obtained by introducing contrast medium either by cannulation of the vasa deferentia through scrotal incisions or by catheterisation of ejaculatory ducts with special urethroscopic equipment.

Matapurkar and Taneja (1969) were able to diagnose cancer in 17 of 20 cases; signs indicating early local spread included narrowing and elongation of ejaculatory ducts, amputation of the ampulla of the vas, and narrowing and irregularity of the seminal vesicles. In another series of patients, five cases with stage T2 disease were considered inoperable because of demonstrable involvement of the vesicles (Aledia 1973).

The main limitations of this technique are the necessity for bilateral scrotal incisions and the requirement of considerable experience for reliable interpretation.

3 Direct Imaging Techniques

3.1 Radionuclide Scanning

The prostate contains a high concentration of zinc (Daniel et al. 1956; Mikac-Devic 1970). Studies have shown that the concentration of this element in the normal prostate and in BPH is similar, but that it decreases in cancer. Others have found low zinc values in BPH and prostatitis (Hoare and Delory 1956).

Gold and Lorber (1970) obtained in vivo and in vitro gamma camera scans in dogs following intravenous injection of ^{69m}Zinc. A high turnover rate of the isotope was found, however, within hepatic tissue.

The first human prostatic scans were reported from Walter Reed General Hospital (Anon 1967). With the aid of ^{69m}Zn citrate or chloride, scans were obtained in a group of eight patients. Though it was believed that less than 10% of the isotope reached the prostate there was little background activity around the prostate.

Other radioactive agents used for prostatic scans include ^{62}Zn (Chisholm et al. 1974), ^{131}I estramustine phosphate and diethylstilboestrol diphosphanate (Szendroi 1973). Images obtained to date have not, however, proved suitable for routine diagnostic purposes.

3.2 Prostatography

Prostatic images may be obtained by introducing contrast medium into the prostate via the rectum (Sugiura and Hasegawa 1969) or transperineally (Raghavaiah 1979). Ipsilateral pelvic lymphatics can also be visualised. Delineation of the whole gland, however, requires injection into both lobes. Such techniques have not yet gained widespread acceptance, because of their invasive nature and the potential risk of infection and pulmonary embolisation.

3.3 Ultrasonography

Development and refinement of ultrasonic techniques over the last 20 years have resulted in their current acceptance in clinical diagnosis. Ultrasound enables imaging of the prostate gland directly and makes it possible to estimate with accuracy the volume of the gland and to demonstrate the various disease processes occurring within the gland.
Ultrasonic techniques for prostatic imaging include (1) transabdominal or suprapubic; (2) perineal; (3) transurethral; and (4) transrectal techniques.

3.3.1 Transabdominal Techniques

The patient is examined with a full bladder by means of conventional grey scale B-mode equipment. A series of longitudinal and transverse cross-sectional images of the prostate is obtained (Fig. 1).
Whittingham and Bishop (1973) carried out ultrasonic estimation of volume of the enlarged prostate, using a simple abdominal approach by approximating the shape of the enlarged prostate to an ellipsoid. Results were compared with those obtained by (a) water displacement with the recovered prostate and (b) weight of the resected specimens converted to volume by assuming a specific gravity of 1,000 for prostatic tissue. The accuracy rates were disappointing, disagreement between ultrasound and the water displacement technique being of the order of 30%.
Miller et al. (1973), on comparing prostatic size determined by digital examination, by analysis of bladder films of IVU, and ultrasound found a close correlation between size determined by ultrasonic scans and volume of resected specimens. Volume estimations were made by measuring the diameter of the gland on the scan which showed the largest area of the prostate.
Similar results have been obtained by Henneberry et al. (1979). Loch et al. (1977) have examined a group of patients by transabdominal ultrasound with a special rating apparatus to analyse echo-amplitude patterns of the prostate parenchyma. Prostatic adenomas and carcinomas were recognisable in 85% of the examined patients and good success rates were claimed for the differentiation of normal from abnormal prostatic tissue. These findings have yet to be substantiated by other workers.
The advantages of transabdominal ultrasound relate to the accurate assessment of prostatic size and to the ease of monitoring effects of chemotherapy in both carcinoma and BPH without any adjustment or addition to basic ultrasound equipment. The major limitations are its poor ability, at present, to characterise disease processes accurately compared with transrectal ultrasound, and the difficulty in examining the obese patient (Fig. 2).

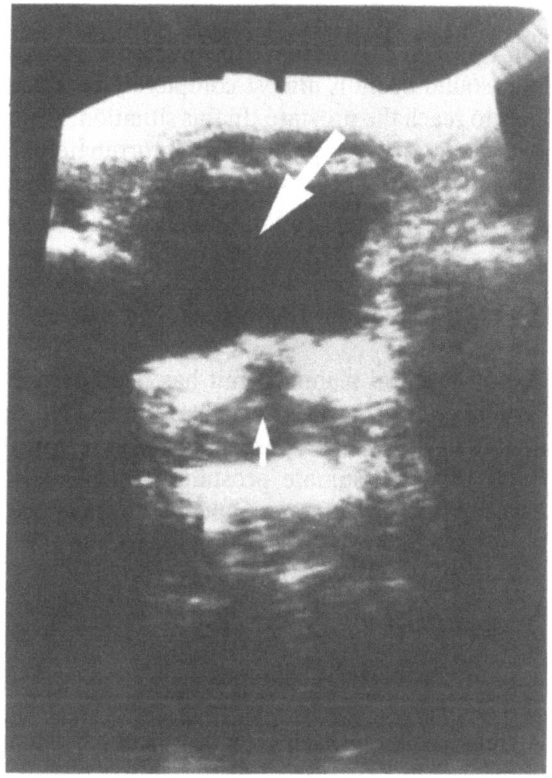

Fig. 1. Transverse transabdominal grey scale B scan. The full bladder (*large arrow*) acts as an acoustic window through which to view the prostate (*small arrow*)

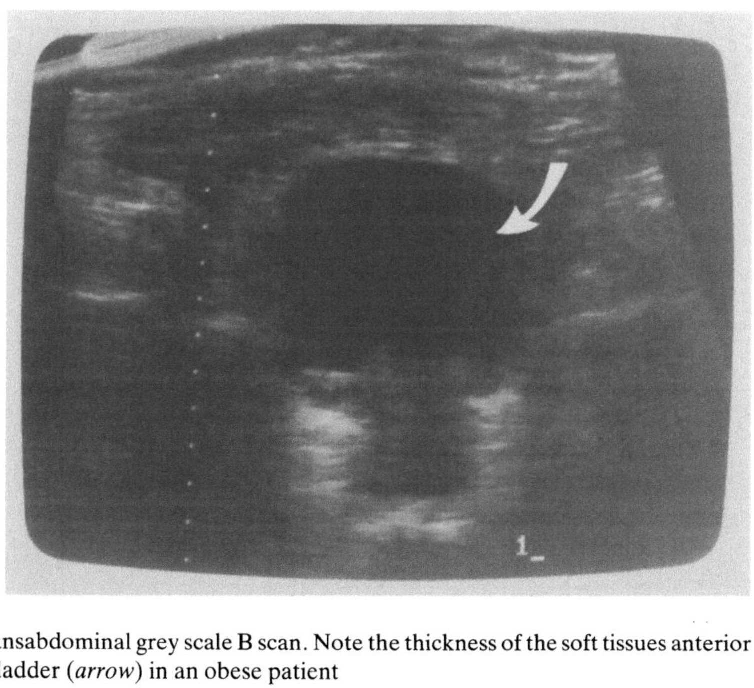

Fig. 2. Transverse transabdominal grey scale B scan. Note the thickness of the soft tissues anterior to the poorly filled bladder (*arrow*) in an obese patient

3.3.2 Perineal Techniques

On occasion it is difficult to image the prostate by the abdominal approach, as the ultrasound beam is almost completely reflected by the pubic bone and consequently fails to reach the prostate. In this situation, it may be possible to demonstrate the gland by scanning via the perineum. Unfortunately, contact is unstable even with the more versatile probe of real time ultrasonic equipment (Emisonic 4500) and the method in our experience has not yet proved entirely successful (Fig. 3).

3.3.3 Transurethral Techniques

A transurethral scanning unit has been described which is interchangeable with the ordinary optics in a cystoscope (Holm and Northved 1974). Transverse cross-sectional images of the prostate perpendicular to the prostatic urethra are produced. As well as being used to estimate prostatic volume and the presence and extent of prostatic cancer, this instrument could well prove to be extremely useful as a guide to transurethral prostatic resection, providing a constant demonstration of the distance to the prostatic capsule during resection.

3.3.4 Transrectal Techniques

A transrectal approach provides the most reliable method of examining the prostate ultrasonically. The use of ultrasound to obtain a cross-sectional pattern of the entire prostate via the rectum was first made by Japanese workers who developed the original

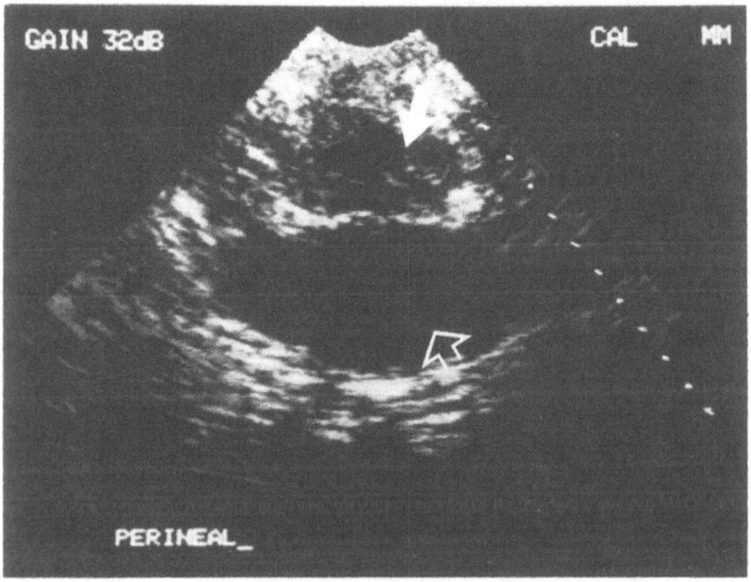

Fig. 3. Sagittal perineal real time sector scan. In this plane the prostate (*closed arrow*) is close to the examining probe and the bladder (*open arrow*) is more distant

equipment in 1967 (Watanabe et al. 1971). Since then a number of reports have originated from the same group, describing their experiences with transrectal sonography.

3.3.5 Technical Considerations

The rectal probe consists of two concentric tubes, an outer stationary unit and a freely moving inner assembly. The transducer is situated at the end of the inner assembly and has a rotating mean frequency of 3.5 mHz. The beam is emitted at right angles to the probe and has a pulse repetition rate of 1,000 per second. The inner tube can move longitudinally and so produce sections of the bladder and prostate at any level. It also rotates to provide sonar tomograms at each of these levels.

Prior to rectal insertion, the outer tube is covered with a disposable rubber balloon. After insertion, the balloon is filled with water until it is air-tight against the rectal mucosa. This not only provides an aqueous interface between the probe and the mucosa, but also serves to protect the mucosal surface.

The patient is in the lithotomy position with his head lowered 15°–20° below the horizontal. The probe is lubricated with a suitable coupling material and passed gently 8–9 cm above the anal verge. Transverse tomograms are obtained through the bladder base and then distally at 0.5-cm intervals through the seminal vesicles and prostate.

In 1974 a new chair type equipment was developed by Watanabe et al. (1975). More recently, grey scale equipment has been used by a number of workers (Boyce et al. 1976; Harada et al. 1979; Peeling et al. 1979) (Fig. 4). Currently a more portable gun-type scanning unit has been introduced, but this has not yet been fully evaluated.

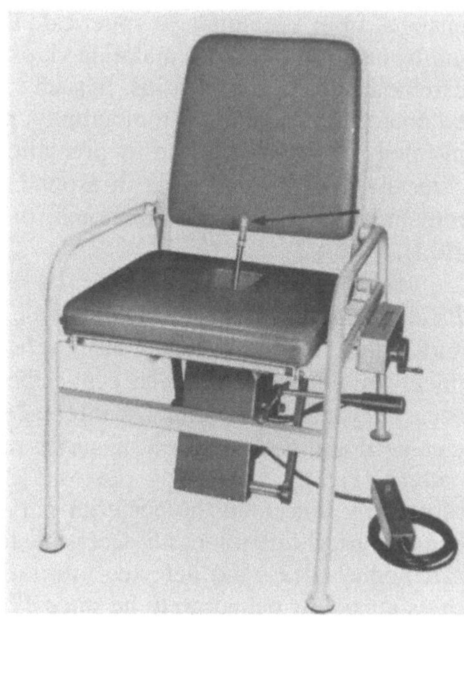

Fig. 4. Chair with adjustable transrectal ultrasound probe

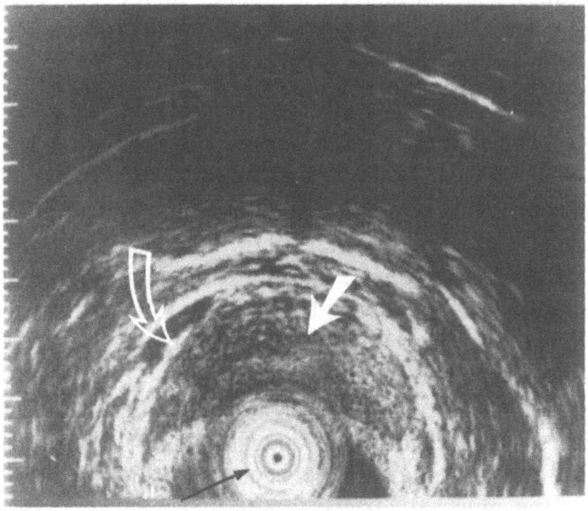

Fig. 5. Ultrasonotomogram with transrectal probe (*black arrow*). Note semilunar shape of the normal prostate (*closed arrow*) with homogeneous internal echo pattern and intact capsule (*open arrow*). Illustration by courtesy of Dr. G. J. Griffiths, Royal Gwent Hospital

3.3.6 Clinical Applications

Normal Prostate (Fig. 1). The normal prostate appears as a well-defined semilunar-shaped organ with its anteroposterior diameter much smaller than the transverse. The clear outline is produced by echoes from the prostatic capsule; within the capsule there is a fine homogeneous echo pattern (Fig. 5).

Benign Prostatic Hyperplasia. There is diffuse enlargement of the gland in BPH, which has its greatest effect on the anteroposterior diameter, so that the shape of the gland changes from semilunar to spherical. Despite the enlargement, the symmetry and uniformity of the gland is maintained, except when there are associated calculi, occult carcinoma, or focal prostatitis. In such cases, with the exception of calculi, which may be detected by computed tomography, pre-operative diagnosis can be made only on histology of tissue removed by prostatic biopsy. In a series of 57 patients with BPH clinically, in only 45 were the ultrasound findings compatible with that diagnosis; in the remainder calculi, occult carcinoma, or normal prostates were found (Boyce et al. 1976).

Prostatic Cancer (Fig. 2). The ultrasonic appearances of cancer are those of distortion and deformity; the capsular echoes become asymmetrical and lose their uniform thickness. Later, the capsular echoes become discontinuous as spread of the disease occurs beyond the capsule. The internal echoes become inhomogeneous, with areas of increased and decreased echogenicity replacing the normal homogeneous fine echo pattern (Fig. 6).
Most early cancers in the posterior part of the gland are readily palpable, but those lying anteriorly are not easily accessible to palpation. In a selected group of 26 cases of carcinoma, ultrasound detected infiltration beyond the capsule in five of the seven cases judged by palpation to be stage T2 tumours (Watanabe et al. 1975). Resnick et

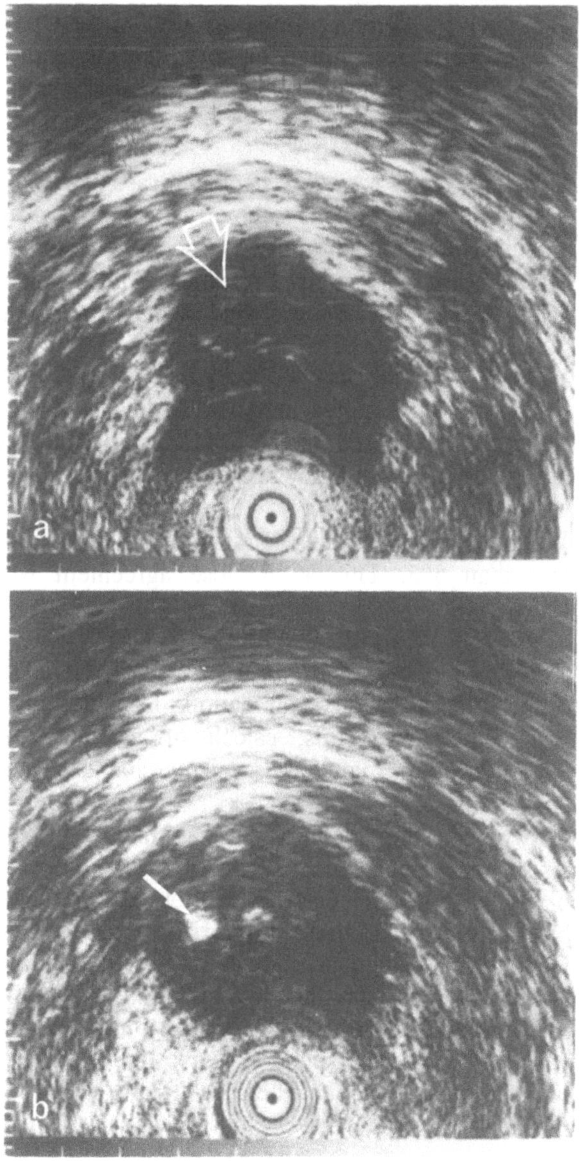

Fig. 6a, b. Transrectal ultrasonotomogram. **a** Advanced carcinoma (*arrow*) with irregular shape and disruption of prostatic capsule; **b** 1 cm caudal to **a**. Note echo-dense areas (*arrow*) suggestive of associated calcification. Illustration by courtesy of Dr. G. J. Griffiths, Royal Gwent Hospital

al. (1977) demonstrated involvement of the seminal vesicles in two out of seven cases with clinical stage T2 cancer.

In a recent British study, ultrasound identified 32 of 33 men with proven cancer; good correlation was found between ultrasound and clinical methods when spread occurred posteriorly or laterally. In almost half the patients with clinically localised disease, however, the disease had spread anteriorly and was not accessible to palpation.

Problems with diagnosis occur when the ultrasonic findings show an area of localised dense echoes within an intact capsule; an early prostatic cancer (T1 and T2) can only be differentiated from inflammatory disease by prostatic biopsy. With more extensive lesions diagnostic accuracy with ultrasound is impressive, but there is still an overall false-negative rate of 23%.

Prostatitis and Prostatic Calculi. Ultrasonically the gland may be normal in size or enlarged, but it remains symmetrical; in prostatitis the capsular echoes may become irregular but their continuity is likely to be maintained, while the internal echo pattern often becomes irregular. Prostatic calculi produce asymmetrical areas of increased echogenicity with acoustic shadowing distal to them.

Assessment of Prostatic Volume. It is possible to calculate prostatic size and volume from dimensions represented on the tomogram. The volume is calculated from the sum of areas represented on the tomograms taken at different levels. Since the specific gravity of prostatic tissue is about 1,000, the volume is about equal to the prostatic weight.
Watanabe (1979) found the range of error in the measurement of prostatic size to be less than 5%. This is in close agreement with the findings of Boyce et al. (1976).

Assessment of the Solitary Prostatic Nodule. Small nodular or indurated areas are often discovered on rectal examination. Benign nodules may be secondary to nodular hyperplasia, prostatitis, calculi or vascular injury. Malignant nodules include adenocarcinoma, squamous cell carcinoma, transitional cell carcinoma, sarcoma, lymphoma, and metastases.
Fifty percent of palpable nodules are malignant (Jewett 1956), and it is not possible to distinguish benign from malignant lesions by rectal examination alone. Perineal needle biopsy has a diagnostic error of about 30% (Kaufman and Schultz 1962). Transrectal biopsy is more accurate but carries a risk of infection.
Benign and malignant nodules present different ultrasonic appearances. The echo pattern from nodules of benign hyperplasia is indistinguishable from the pattern of the surrounding hyperplastic gland. Malignant nodules give rise to irregular dense echoes which attenuate the sound and give rise to acoustic shadowing beyond them. If the tumour is large enough, the capsule may be distorted or broken and spread into the periprostatic tissue may be observed.

Mass Screening Programmes. A mass screening survey has been carried out in a group of asymptomatic men within the age range 40–76 years (Watanabe et al. 1977). Of a total of 132 men examined, 48 patients underwent secondary studies, including prostatic biopsy. Eighteen patients had BPH, half of them having clinical indications for prostatectomy. No unsuspected malignancy was detected.
Further studies are necessary before this ultrasonic technique can be used on a routine basis both for diagnostic imaging and screening programmes.

Diagnostic Accuracy. The accuracy rates for bistable and grey scale equipment for various prostatic diseases are shown in Table 2. Table 3 shows the false-negative and false-positive rates with various methods used for the diagnosis of prostatic cancer.

Table 2. Diagnostic accuracy in prostatic disease[a]

	Bistable (%)	Grey scale (%)
Benign hyperplasia	89	91
Carcinoma	77	85
Prostatitis	66	89
Normal	74	–

[a] Data from Watanabe et al. (1979) and Harada et al. (1979)

Table 3. Diagnostic accuracy in prostatic cancer[a]

	False-negative (%)	False-positive (%)
Rectal palpation	36	30
Urethrography	57	27
Acid phosphatase	66	58
Needle biopsy	24	38
Ultrasound	23	26

[a] Data from Watanabe et al. (1975)

3.4 Computed Tomography (CT)

The ability of computed tomography to discriminate small changes in density has provided a useful method for imaging the abdominal and pelvic viscera. In the pelvis, CT often provides adequate demonstration of the viscera and surrounding fat, muscles, and bony pelvic walls. Nevertheless, experience with CT scanning of the pelvis and the prostate in particular is limited, and to date only a single small comparative study with transabdominal ultrasound has been reported (Sukov et al. 1977).

3.4.1 Technical Considerations

All patients in our own centre receive bowel preparation for 48 h (Isogel 10 ml twice daily) and oral water-soluble contrast (Gastrografin 250 ml 5%) 12 h, 90 min, and 30 min before the examination. Bowel paralysis with anticholinergic drugs is contraindicated and not essential in this group of patients. A bolus dose of intravenous contrast (40 ml Conray 280) is administered before commencing the examination. In patients with a drainage catheter in situ, a double-contrast CT cystogram is performed by introducing a maximum of 150 ml air after the contrast is injected intravenously.

The pelvis is scanned from the level of the anterior superior iliac spines at 2-cm intervals to the level of the bladder fundus and at 1-cm intervals thereafter. Sections are taken in the 20-s mode except those through the prostate when the 70-s mode is used to improve density discrimination.

3.4.2 Diagnostic Limitations

Unopacified Bowel Loops. Unopacified bowel often cannot be distinguished from abnormal masses with certainty. In these circumstances it is necessary to examine contiguous sections closely. Unopacified bowel loops will be shown to be continuous with contrast-filled segments. Interrogation at narrower window widths often shows some contrast or air. Occasionally it may be necessary to repeat the examination after giving larger oral doses of contrast medium.
The rectum is often identified without much difficulty, but in some cases administration of rectal contrast medium or inflation of a balloon catheter is helpful.

Tissue Characterisation. Despite the ability of CT in some circumstances to distinguish heterogeneity of composition of tissue, reliable histological characterisation is not yet available. Several approaches to tissue characterisation are currently being investigated but all have significant constraints.

Angiography implies visualisation of the intra- and extravascular spaces of an organ after rapid intravenous injection of contrast medium. Temporal changes in contrast enhancement may provide additional information. Precise positioning and accurate reproducibility of thin body sections in all spatial co-ordinates does, however, present significant problems.

Tomochemistry. The feasibility of extracting the electron density and effective atomic number of tissue from measurements of attenuation values at different beam energies has previously been reported (Rutherford et al. 1976). The method is subject to certain intrinsic limitations relating to accuracy, sensitivity, and the relevance of chemical changes encountered in disease (Isherwood et al. 1977).

Analysis of Distribution of Attenuation Values. Attenuation values measured by CT are distributed in both magnitude and space. Distribution in magnitude can be described by a histogram. Other parameters, including analysis of gradients and the autocorrelation function, are required to describe spatial distribution (Ritchings et al. 1979).

Boundary Definition. Accurate boundary definition is important when measurements are made on the CT images. Boundary definition often depends upon window settings, the amount of fat between surrounding organs, and the partial volume effect. Clear differentiation of the prostate from the levator ani muscles and the rectum is often difficult because of lack of fat (Van Engelshoven and Kreel 1979).

Anatomical Considerations. The prostate is usually visualised in sections obtained through the symphysis pubis as an ovoid density at the bladder base. The normal prostate has a smooth outline and appears of homogeneous density (Fig. 7). The prostatic capsule, parenchyma, and venous plexus cannot normally be differentiated. In the ischiorectal fossae the inferior rectal vessels may be seen occasionally. The dorsal vein of the penis and the obturator vessels may also be identified.
The seminal vesicles are of variable thickness and form an angle, the seminal vesicle angle, with the posterior aspect of the bladder (Fig. 8). These structures may exhibit

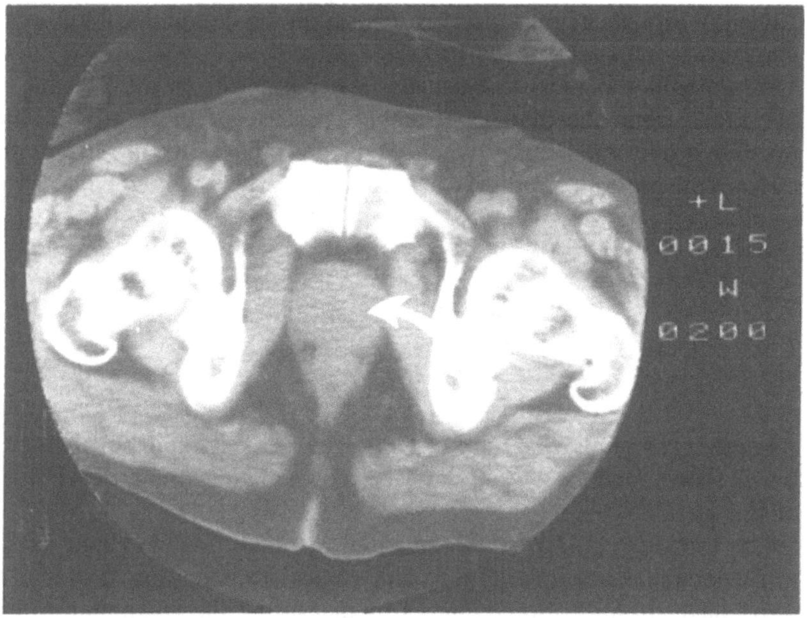

Fig. 7. CT scan of normal prostate. Note smooth outline and homogeneous density. The posterior margin of the prostate is not clearly distinguished from the rectum

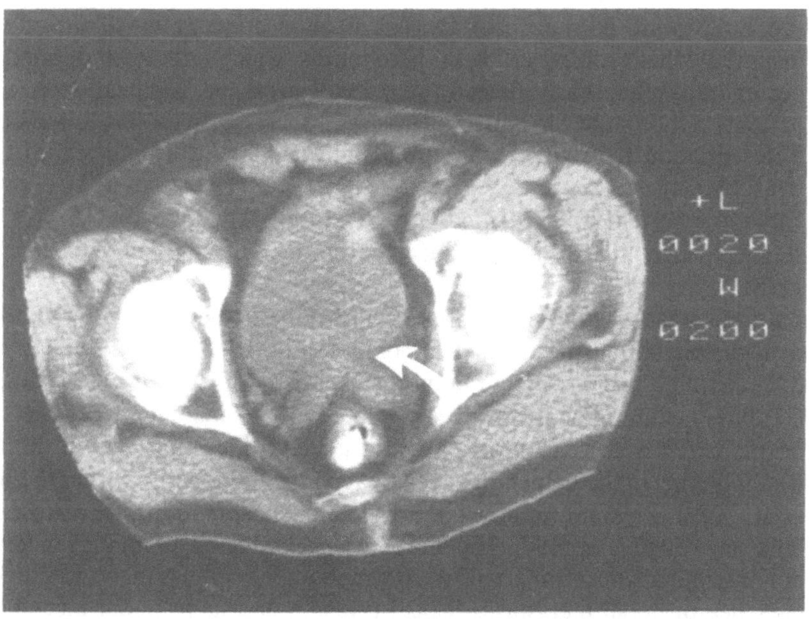

Fig. 8. CT scan of normal seminal vesicle angle (*arrow*). Note left inguinal lymphadenopathy due to metastatic spread from prostatic carcinoma

considerable mobility with difference in position of the patient. The seminal vesicle angle, in normal circumstances, is reduced in the lateral decubitus position and often abolished completely in the prone position.

The urine-filled bladder can usually be separated from the prostate, but difficulties may arise when the bladder is empty, because of the partial volume effect. The prostate is better delineated when the bladder fills with contrast; contrast often leaks out into the prostatic urethra, which is then clearly visualised lying centrally within the gland.

3.4.3 Clinical Applications

Assessment of Shape, Size, and Volume. The gross size and morphology of the prostate is well shown, and focal lesions may be shown as an asymmetrical bulge in the contour of the gland.

Sukov et al. (1977) have compared estimations of gland size obtained by transabdominal ultrasound, CT, and clinical examination. Volume determinations were made from ultrasonic images by measuring the maximum AP, transverse and supero-inferior dimensions and calculating the volume of an equivalent sphere. From the CT images, volume was calculated from the AP and transverse diameters from the section having the largest cross-sectional area. Ultrasound was more accurate than clinical examination and CT, which tended to overemphasize the gland size. This is not surprising in view of the problems with boundary definition mentioned above.

Detection of Calculi and Differentiation from Phleboliths. Because of the sensitivity of CT, foci of calcification and calculi are usually well shown when conventional plain radiographs are normal; prostatic calcification appears irregular and more centrally disposed when compared with phleboliths which are well defined and situated peripherally. The early detection of small areas of calcification is useful in those patients who show localised areas of dense echoes on ultrasound, enabling differentiation from other conditions with similar ultrasonic features (Fig. 9).

Staging and Radiotherapy Planning. A more useful role of CT may be in tumour staging, where it may help reduce the number of cases understaged (Levitt et al. 1978).

Lateral spread of tumour into the periprostatic tissues is seen on CT as a soft-tissue density, disrupting the normal fat planes (Fig. 10). Enlarged pelvic nodes may be demonstrated and associated bony metastases outlined (Fig. 11). Tumour staging by CT has its limitations, however, because of its inability to detect metastases in normal-sized nodes. Experience with bladder cancer has shown that CT has been disappointing in the detection of regional lymphadenopathy within the pelvis (Hodson et al. 1979). Prostatic cancer with no detectable spread into periprostatic tissue may have microscopic spread. The most accurate staging of malignancies may require pelvic lymphadenectomy, since even lymphangiography is inaccurate in evaluating the presence of nodal metastases. Local invasion and large nodal metastases, however, will often be detected. Extracapsular spread may result in widening or filling in of the seminal vesicle angle (Seidelmann et al. 1977).

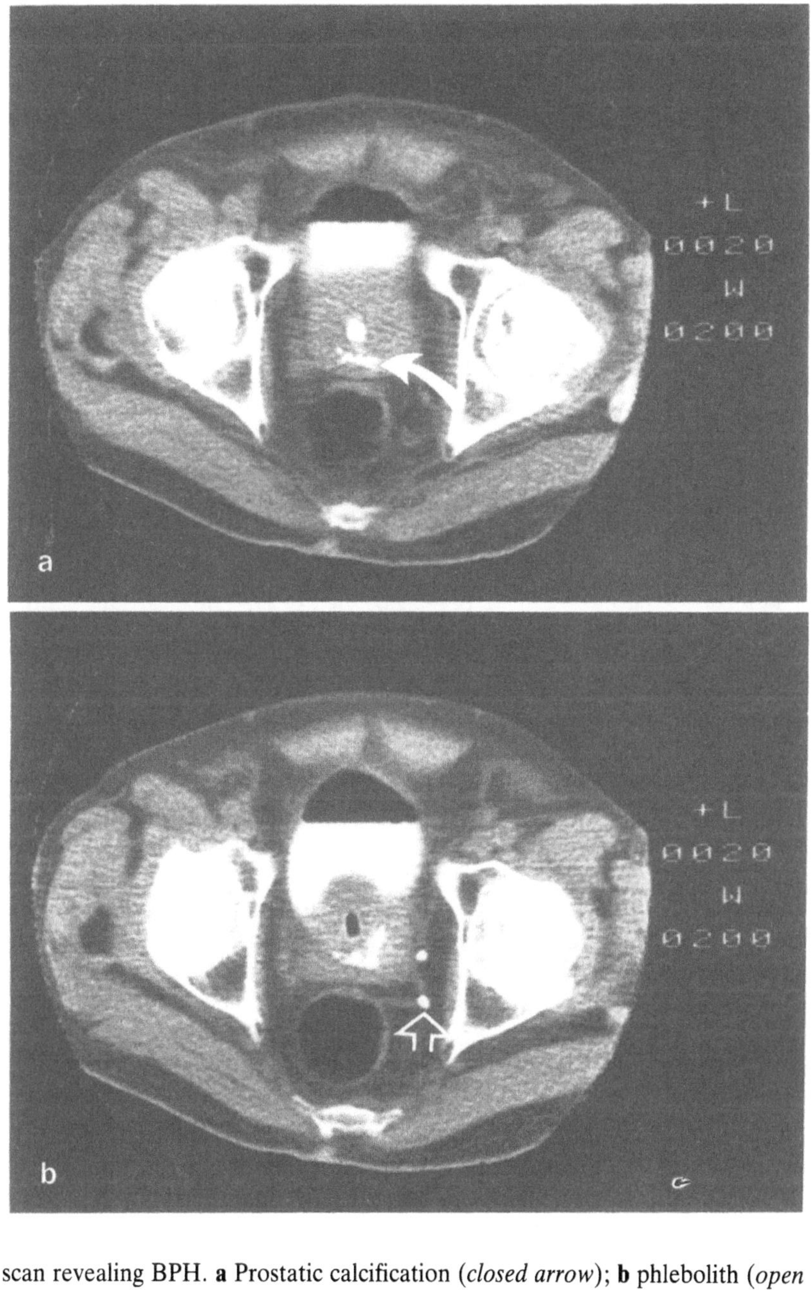

Fig. 9a, b. CT scan revealing BPH. **a** Prostatic calcification (*closed arrow*); **b** phlebolith (*open arrow*)

Recently, Brizel et al. (1979) undertook a prospective study to evaluate the usefulness of CT for radiotherapy management and treatment planning of various pelvic malignancies, including prostatic cancer. All diagnoses were established surgically prior to referral for radiotherapy. The CT findings were compared with operative findings, clinical and routine radiographic findings, and results of pathological examination.

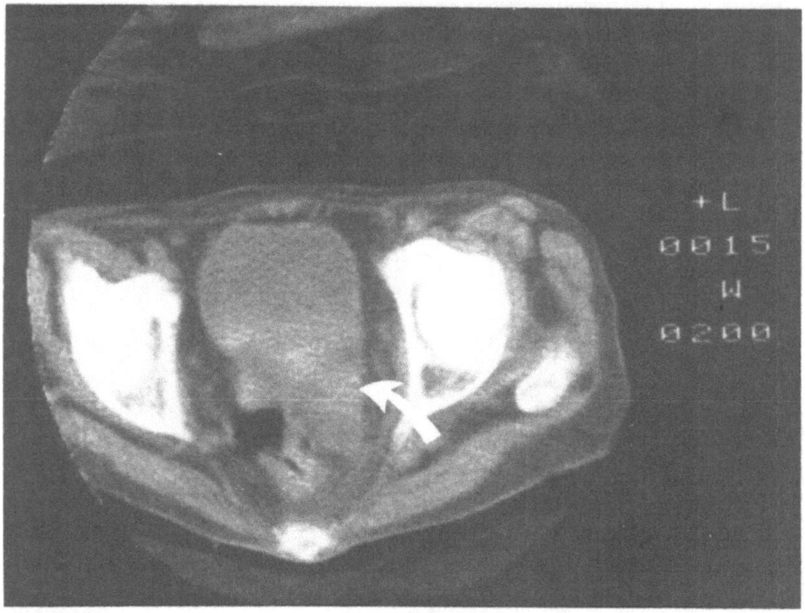

Fig. 10. CT scan revealing prostatic carcinoma. Note extensive left periprostatic spread (*arrow*)

Of 14 patients, CT demonstrated the prostate to be of unanticipated dimensions in six. Extraprostatic spread was demonstrated in five of seven patients in whom tumour was thought to be confined within the capsule. These changes in tumour size and extension resulted in upstaging of four patients.

Although CT cannot in some circumstances distinguish normal from tumour tissue, involvement of seminal vesicles, periprostatic invasion or invasion of the bladder wall may result in upstaging of the growth from intra- to extracapsular disease. In such cases, radiotherapy field arrangements are likely to be significantly modified. Overall clinical assessment without CT underestimated size and extent of tumour in nearly half of the patients.

Assessment of Response to Treatment. Computed tomography offers a simple, non-invasive method for assessing response to treatment. In the study by Brizel et al. (1979) CT allowed further changes in therapy, such as additional booster therapy or addition of unplanned surgery or chemotherapy. Serial measurements of prostatic size are also of value in following the progress and response to treatment of patients with BPH and acute inflammatory conditions. The role of CT in this area has as yet not been explored.

CT is unlikely to replace transrectal ultrasonography as the primary direct imaging technique of choice but occasions when it may be useful include (i) when ultrasound is indeterminate or images are poor, for example in obese patients; (ii) when intracapsular carcinoma is suspected on ultrasound but differentiation from calcification, which may have similar appearances, is necessary; (iii) in the assessment of extent of malignancy and radiotherapy treatment planning together with the monitoring of response to treatment.

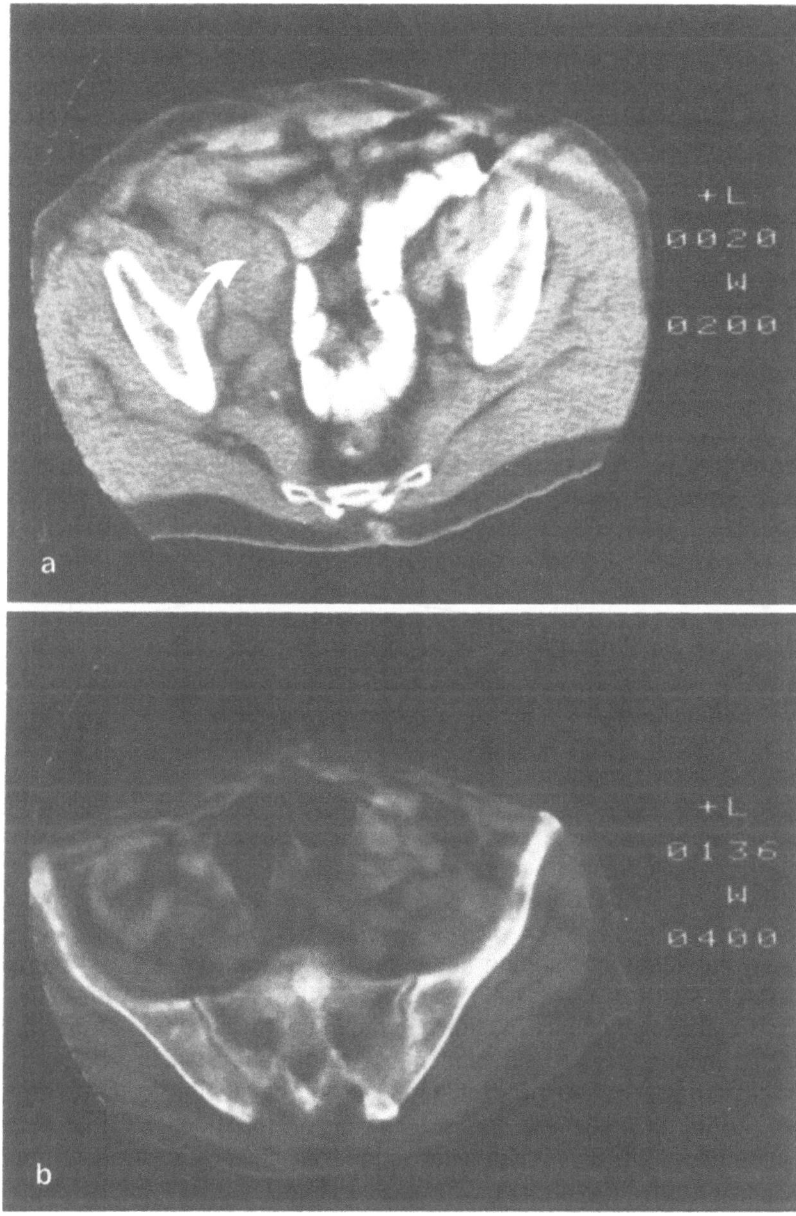

Fig. 11a, b. CT scan revealing prostatic carcinoma. **a** External iliac lymph node metastases (*arrow*). Note value of opacifying small bowel; **b** bony metastases

4 Conclusion

Ultrasound and CT are likely to alter the approach to management of patients with prostatic disease significantly, prostatic cancer in particular. While the precise role of the IVU remains to be defined, it is likely to remain at present in the management

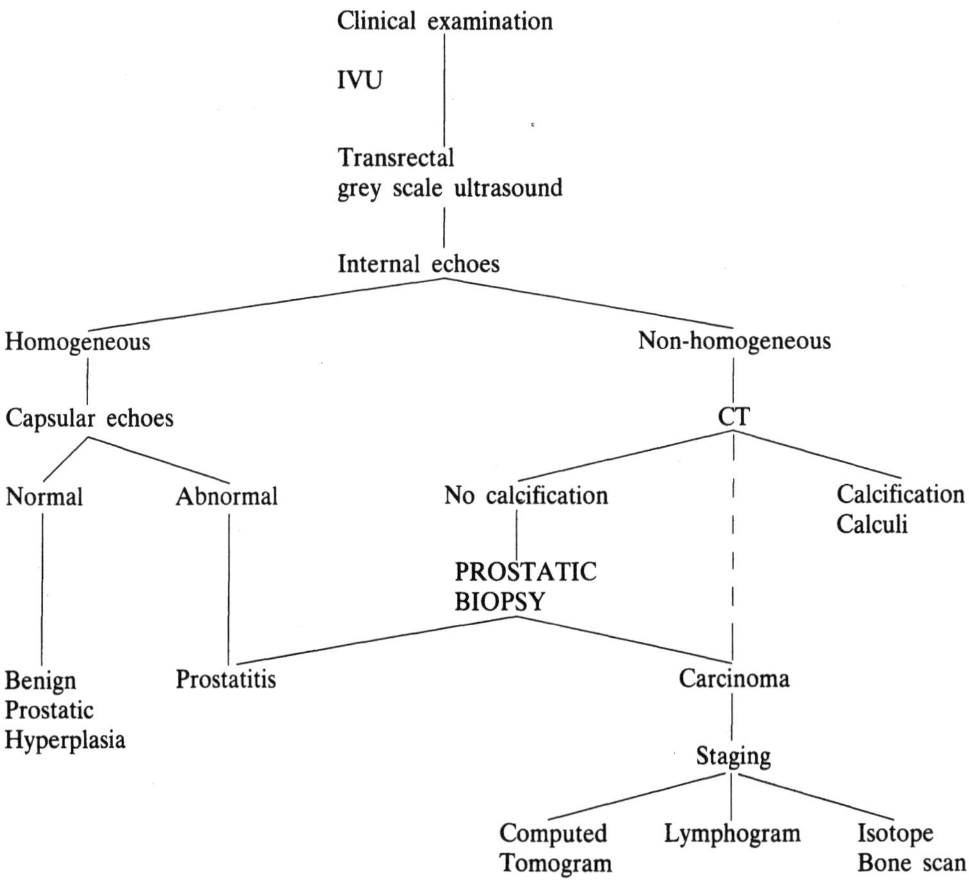

Fig. 12. Diagnostic strategy for prostatic disease

plan, providing information about the upper urinary tract and indirect evidence of prostatic disease. Grey scale transrectal ultrasound should form the direct non-invasive imaging modality of choice in the initial investigation of prostatic disease, with CT providing useful supplementary information when there is doubt, where calcification needs to be excluded, and in the staging, radiotherapy planning and monitoring of malignant disease. The main limitation of CT at present is its poor performance at tissue characterisation. A diagnostic strategy for patients with suspected prostatic disease is proposed (Fig. 12).

5 References

Abrams PH, Roylance J, Feneley RCL (1968) Excretion urography in the investigation of prostatism. Br J Urol 48: 681–684

Abrams PH, Farrar DJ, Turner-Warwick RT, Whiteside CG, Feneley RCL (1979) The results of prostatectomy: A symptomatic and urodynamic analysis of 152 patients. J Urol 121: 640–642

Aledia FT (1973) Vaso-seminal vesiculography: A diagnostic aid in early metastatic carcinoma of prostate. J Urol 110: 242–244

Anonymous (1967) Prostatic scans. JAMA 200: 19 (editorial)
Belli I, Porro RC, Favero CD, Nascimbene C, Tenti L (1978) Lo studio radiologico delle affezioni della prostata. Radiol Med (Torino) 64: 769–784
Blacklock NJ (1977) Prostatic cancer. Urol Res 5: 1–5
Bobbio A, Bezzi E, Rossi L (1959) Pelvic angiography in diseases of prostate gland. AJR 82: 784–792
Boerema WJ (1972) Intravenous pyelography before prostatectomy: An evolution of its use. Aust NZ J Surg 42: 35–38
Boyce WH, McKinney WM, Resnick MI, Willard JW (1976) Ultrasonography as an aid in the diagnosis and management of surgical disease of the pelvis. Ann Surg 184: 477–489
Brizel HE, Livingston PA, Grayson EV (1979) Radiotherapeutic applications of pelvic computed tomography. Journal of Computer-assisted Tomography 3: 453–466
Chisholm GD, Short MD, Ghanadian R, McRae CU, Glass HI (1974) Radiozinc uptake and scintiscanning in prostatic disease. J Nucl Med 15: 739–742
Daniel O, Haddad P, Prout G, Whitmore WF (1956) Some observations on the distribution of radioactive zinc in prostatic and other human tissues. Br J Urol 28: 271–278
Goerttler U (1977) Prostata-Arteriographie, Gefäßversorgung, Diagnose und Differentialdiagnose des Prostata-Adenoma und Carcinoms. Radiologe 17: 256–262
Gold GM, Lorber SA (1970) Radio-isotope ^{69m}Zn chloride prostate gland scan. Invest Urol 8: 231–238
Griffiths HJL, Castro J (1970) An evaluation of the importance of residual urine. Br Radiol 43: 409–413
Harada K, Igari D, Tanahashi Y (1979) Grey scale transrectal ultrasonography of the prostate. Journal of Clinical Ultrasound 7: 45–49
Henneberry M, Carter MF, Newman HL (1979) Estimation of prostatic size by suprapubic ultrasonography. J Urol 121: 615–616
Hoare R, Delory GE (1956) Zinc and acid phosphatase in human prostate. Cancer 9: 721–726
Hodson NJ, Husband E, Macdonald S (1979) The role of computed tomography in the staging of bladder cancer. Clin Radiol 30: 389–395
Holm HH, Northved A (1974) A trans-urethral ultrasonic scanner. J Urol 3: 238–241
Isherwood I, Pullan BR, Rutherford RA, Strang FA (1977) Electron density and atomic number determination by computed tomography. Br J Radiol 50: 613–619
Jewett JH (1956) Significance of the palpable prostatic nodule. JAMA 160 (10): 838–839
Kaufman J, Schultz J (1962) Needle biopsy of the prostate – a re-evaluation. J Urol 87: 164
King WW, Wilkiemeyer RM, Boyce WH, McKinney WM (1973) Current status of prostatic echography. JAMA 226: 444–447
Laubenberger T, Berghaus H (1966) The roentgen exploration of the prostate and urinary bladder floor veins. Peri-prostatic phlebography – a new method. Am J Roentgenol 98: 209–214
Levitt RG, Sage SS, Stanely RJ, Evens RG (1978) Computed tomography of the pelvis. Semin Roentgenol 13: 193–203
Loch EG, Gaca A, Wessels G (1977) Ultraschalluntersuchungen der Prostata mit Datengeräten zur Erkennung von Tumorerkrankungen. Radiologe 16: 356–359
McCallum RW, Colapinto V (1970) In: Urological radiology of the adult male lower urinary tract. Chas. C. Thomas, Springfield, Illinois, pp 98–106
Marshall V, Singh M, Blandy JP (1975) Is urography necessary for patients with acute retention of urine before prostatectomy? Br J Urol 47: 73–76
Matapurkar BG, Taneja OP (1969) A critical evaluation of vaso-seminal vesiculography. Br J Urol 41: 455
Mikac-Devic D (1970) Zinc determinations in biochemical processes. Adv Clin Chem 13: 271–333

Miller SS, Garvie WHH, Christie AD (1973) The evaluation of prostate size by ultrasonic scanning – a preliminary report. Br J Urol 45: 187–191
Peeling WB, Griffiths GJ, Evans KT, Roberts EE (1979) Diagnosis and staging of prostatic cancer by transrectal ultrasonography – a preliminary study. Br J Urol 51: 565–569
Raghavaiah NV (1979) Prostatography. J Urol 121: 174–177
Resnick MI, Willard JW, Boyce WH (1977) Recent progress in ultrasonography of bladder and prostate. J Urol 117: 444–446
Resnick MI, Willard JW, Boyce WH (1978) Ultrasonic evaluation of the prostatic nodule. J Urol 120: 86–89
Ritchings RT, Pullan BR, Lucas SB, Fawcitt RA, Best JJK, Isherwood I, Morris AI (1979) An analysis of the spatial distribution of attenuation values in computed tomographic liver and spleen scans. Journal of Computer-assisted Tomography 3: 36–39
Rutherford RA, Pullan BR, Isherwood I (1976) Measurement of effective atomic number and electron density using an EMI scanner. Neuroradiology 11: 15–21
Seidelmann FE, Reich NW, Cotton WE (1977) Computed tomography of the seminal vesicle and seminal vesicle angle. Computerized Tomography 1: 79–84
Sugiura H, Hasegawa S (1969) Transrectal prostatography – its use in prostatic hypertrophy. Am J Roentgenol 107: 796–802
Sukov RJ, Scardino PT, Sample WF, Winter J, Confer DJ (1977) Computed tomography and transabdominal ultrasound in the evaluation of the prostate. Journal of Computer-assisted Tomography 1: 281–289
Szendroi Z (1973) Isotope scanning of the prostate. Lancet 1: 1252–1253
Thumann RC Jr (1951) Estimation of weight of hyperplastic prostate from cystourethrogram. Am J Roentgenol 65: 593–595
Turner-Warwick R (1973) A urodynamic view of prostatic obstruction and the results of prostectomy. Br J Urol 45: 631–645
Van Engelshoven JMA, Kreel L (1979) Computed tomography of the prostate. Journal of Computer-assisted Tomography 3: 45–51
Vermooten V, Schweinsberg M (1964) Radiographic estimation of size of the prostate. Radiology 86: 1010–1015
Watanabe H (1979) Prostatic ultrasound. In: Rosenfield AT (ed) Genito-urinary ultrasonography. Churchill Livingstone, Edinburgh (Clinics in diagnostic ultrasound, vol 2)
Watanabe H, Igari D, Tanahashi Y, Harada K, Saitoh M (1975) Transrectal ultrasonotomography of the prostate. J Urol 114: 734–739
Watanabe H, Kaiho H, Tanaka M, Terasawa Y (1971) Diagnostic application of ultrasonotomography to the prostate. Invest Urol 8: 548–559
Watanabe H, Saitoh M, Igari D, Mishina T, Tanahashi Y, Harada K, Hisamichi S (1977) Mass screening program for prostatic diseases with transrectal ultrasonotomography. J Urol 117: 746–748
Whittingham TA, Bishop R (1973) Ultrasonic estimation of the enlarged prostate. Br J Radiol 46: 68–70

Lymphography

J. S. Macdonald

Department of Diagnostic Radiology, Royal Marsden Hospital, Institute of Cancer Research, GB – London

1 Introduction

In carcinoma of the prostate, involvement of regional lymph nodes can occur early in its natural history and be independent of haematogenous spread, as demonstrated by Flocks et al. (1959) in a surgical series of 411 patients. The significance of lymph node involvement in treatment strategy and its importance in prognosis is considerable (Flocks 1973).

Hilaris et al. (1977) found in 208 patients who had bilateral pelvic lymphadenectomy that all those with stage T1–3 tumours and negative nodes were disease-free at 5 years. Of the patients with T4 tumours and negative nodes, or T1–2 tumours and positive nodes, 90% were alive at 5 years, although 30% had distant metastases. Of those with T3–4 tumours and positive nodes, 70% were alive at 5 years, 50% of whom had distant metastases. There is therefore little argument about the prognostic significance of lymph node involvement.

How effectively can lymph node metastases be demonstrated by radiological techniques? Lymphography is a direct radiological method of opacifying some parts of the lymphatic system, and this chapter is concerned with its limitations and its applications in patients with carcinoma of the prostate.

2 Limitations

Lymphography from the feet does not opacify the obturator nodes and therefore these are not shown. This has to be considered by the radiotherapist when planning radiation treatment. Lymphography will only pick up metastases when they have reached the iliac nodes and of course when they have passed beyond these to the para-aortic region.

There is also the failure rate of the technique to consider. Technical failure to cannulate the lymphatics will be encountered in 1% or 2% of patients. Carcinoma of the prostate occurs in older patients, who may have a poor respiratory reserve, and a proportion of these will be considered unsuitable for lymphography; such cases must also be taken as failures of lymphography. Patient selection and complications in lymphography have been considered elsewhere (Macdonald 1976). It is enough to say that lymphography is a safe and reliable technique in experienced hands, provided that too much contrast medium is not injected and those with already impaired lung function are not subjected to excessive pulmonary oil embolism.

Recent Results in Cancer Research, Vol. 78
© Springer-Verlag Berlin · Heidelberg 1981

3 Diagnostic Accuracy

O'Donoghue et al. (1976) stated: "However, the accuracy of lymphography in the detection of nodal metastases continues to be a source of controversy in many tumour sites." They then described their experience in a series of 20 patients where lymphography was compared with findings at lymphadenectomy. Three patients had positive lymphograms, and one of these was found to be a false-positive. Seventeen were negative at lymphography, and three of these were positive histologically, i.e., false-negative. The overall accuracy of this series was therefore 75%. But the only definite criterion for deposits which they used was that there should be filling defects larger than 5 mm in diameter in the nodes.

Spellman et al. (1977) evaluated the accuracy of lymphography in previously untreated patients with carcinoma of the prostate, using laparotomy and selective lymph node biopsy. This was a prospective trial with carefully controlled biopsy and an accuracy rate of 78%. But the only criterion which they used for diagnosing involved nodes was that a filling defect should be more than 10 mm in diameter. They did not find para-aortic nodes involved without evidence of lymph node involvement in the pelvis.

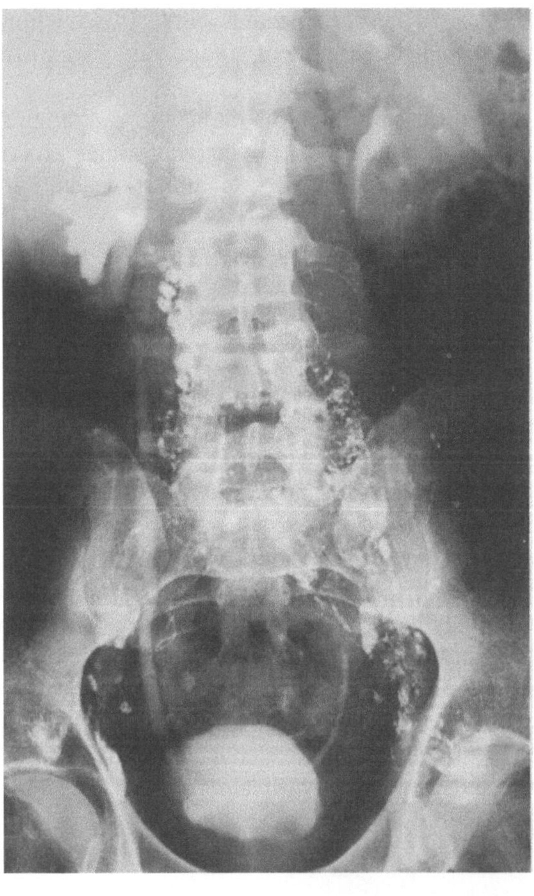

Fig. 1. Patient with carcinoma of the prostate, stage T3. Lymphogram (*AP view*) shows grossly involved nodes in both para-aortic and common iliac regions and in the left side of the pelvis. There is stasis in the lymphatics and opening up of collateral channels

Their conclusions were that a 'positive' lymphogram should be considered highly suggestive of metastatic disease but that a 'negative' lymphogram should not be accepted as excluding possible involvement.

Hilaris et al. (1977) reported that lymphography had been performed in 139 of their 208 patients, with an accuracy of 69% when the findings were compared with the results of bilateral pelvic lymphadenectomy. They did not give their diagnostic criteria for lymphography.

These three series reported accuracy rates of 75%, 78%, and 69%, respectively, but it is probable that accuracy could be improved by use of more stringent diagnostic criteria. Measurement of the size of filling defects in opacified nodes and reliance on an arbitrary figure above which a node will be considered to be involved must be unsatisfactory. All deposits begin as a microscopic collection of cells before enlarging, and therefore a deposit cannot be determined by size alone. Also in these reported series, the lymphogram was being used as a 'one-look' examination, a decision being taken on the appearances of the immediate and 24-h radiographs. From our own experience we have found that if these appearances alone are relied on , depending on the tumour type there is an inherent inaccuracy of between 5% and 20%. It is therefore important to consider the diagnostic criteria which should be used in lymphography.

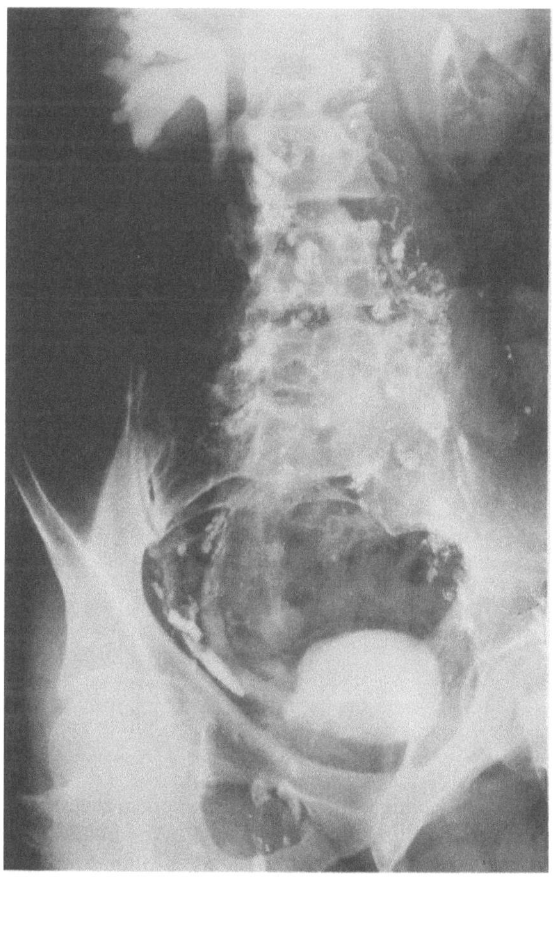

Fig. 2. Same patient as in Fig. 1. Lymphogram (*oblique view*) shows the involved nodes, which are spherical or ellipsoid in shape; this can be assessed by comparing the two projections

4 Diagnostic Criteria of Metastatic Involvement

Figures 1 and 2 show the lymphographic appearances at 24-h in a patient with a T3 carcinoma of the prostate and grossly involved nodes in both para-aortic and in both common iliac regions and on the left side of the pelvis. There is no problem in the diagnosis of positive nodes when they are as grossly involved as these. It is interesting to note the rather untidy appearance of the lymphogram, with stasis and the opening up of many collateral channels. Just as certain types of tumour tend to produce certain patterns of metastates to the lung and to bone, deposits from carcinoma of the prostate and the bladder tend to produce rather messy-looking lymphograms when the nodes are involved. This appearance is probably associated with the slow rate of growth. It should be noted that the involved nodes appear circular in two radiographic projections, the PA and the oblique views. As a deposit grows in a node it progressively enlarges, forming a sphere or an ellipsoid. Deposits in nodes do not grow as flat sheets, so that if a filling defect in a node appears round or oval in two different projections it is much more likely to be a deposit.
Figure 3 shows the appearances in the same patient 6 weeks later, following irradiation. The involved nodes have shown a rapid reduction in size, while the normal

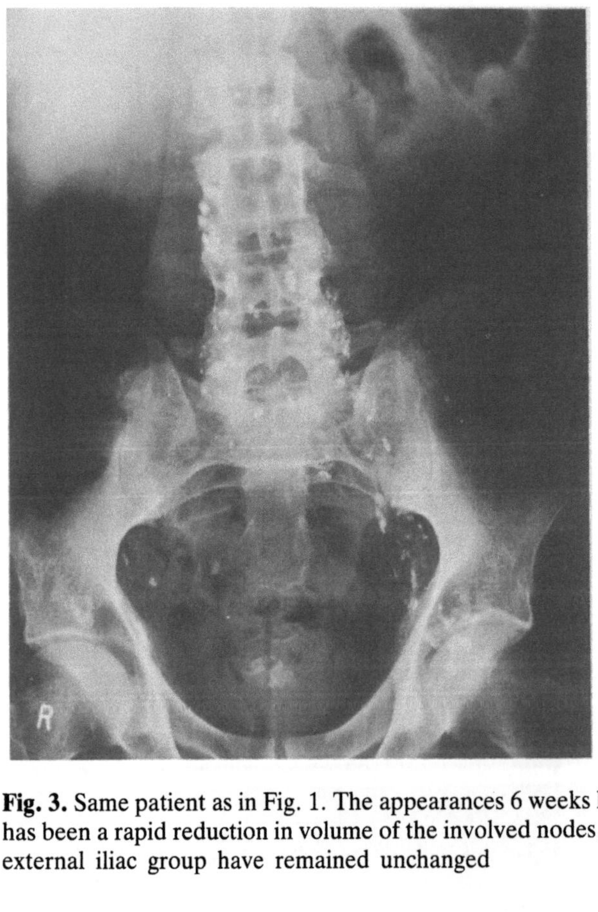

Fig. 3. Same patient as in Fig. 1. The appearances 6 weeks later, following radiotherapy. There has been a rapid reduction in volume of the involved nodes, while the normal nodes in the right external iliac group have remained unchanged

nodes on the right side of the pelvis are unchanged apart from some loss of contrast medium. Figure 4 shows the same patient 6 months later. It is difficult at this stage to pick out an abnormal node. This was a grossly positive lymphogram; there was no problem in diagnosing it as such, but it does illustrate several principles of diagnostic importance:

1) When deposits grow in nodes they tend to be spherical or ellipsoidal in shape.
2) After lymphography the contrast medium is retained in the nodes over a long period (for about a year in diagnostic amounts), and this allows their behaviour to be observed over time.
3) Lymphography should therefore be looked upon as a dynamic investigation.

If follow-up films are not studied, the accuracy of the investigation is reduced, information may be lost about the subsequent behaviour of nodes under treatment, and early spread to other areas may be missed.

Much has been written on the diagnosis of deposits based on the appearances of filling defects in opacified nodes, but this concept has to be taken further. Size itself, unless very large, is of little help, because deposits can be of any size. However, because of

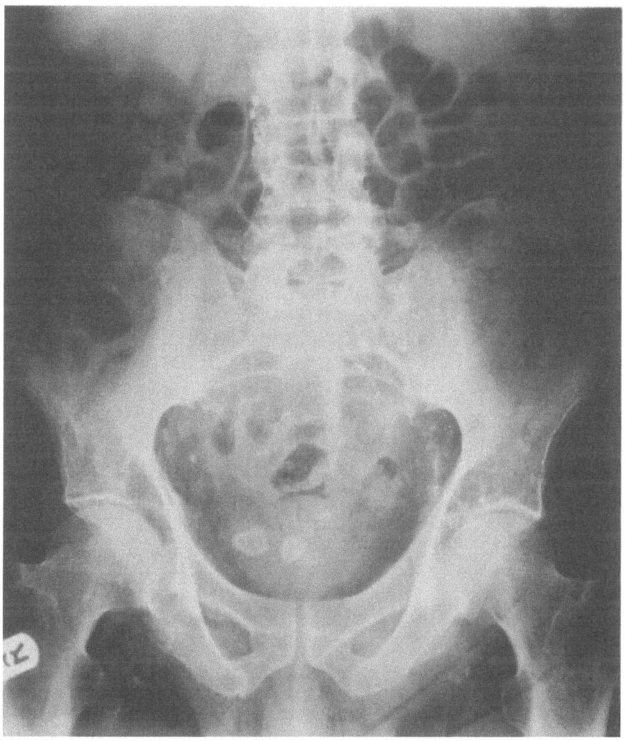

Fig. 4. Same patient as in Fig. 1. Six months later, the treated, involved nodes are now normal in size. Two bladder calculi are present

the way in which deposits grow, which has been described above, the question which should always be in the diagnostic radiologist's mind is not whether or not a well-defined filling defect is present, but rather: 'Do any of the filling defects *look like* and *behave like* expanding lesions?'

In Fig. 5 grossly involved nodes are seen in both sides of the pelvis, particularly on the left, and the para-aortic nodes are suspicious. Following radiotherapy the appearances were as in Fig. 6. The definitely involved nodes have reduced dramatically in size, whereas the doubtful nodes in the para-aortic regions have lost contrast medium, but on measurement are hardly altered. The para-aortic nodes have behaved normally while the involved nodes have contracted dramatically, confirming by their behaviour that they were in fact involved. One group has behaved like nodes affected by cancer, while the other group, although containing filling defects, had behaved normally, which brings out another principle: Cancer should only be diagnosed when it not only looks like cancer, but behaves like cancer.

A great many nodes opacify at each lymphogram and among these there will be groups of normal nodes. The behaviour of these nodes should be used as a control, and any nodes which behave differently should be looked upon with suspicion.

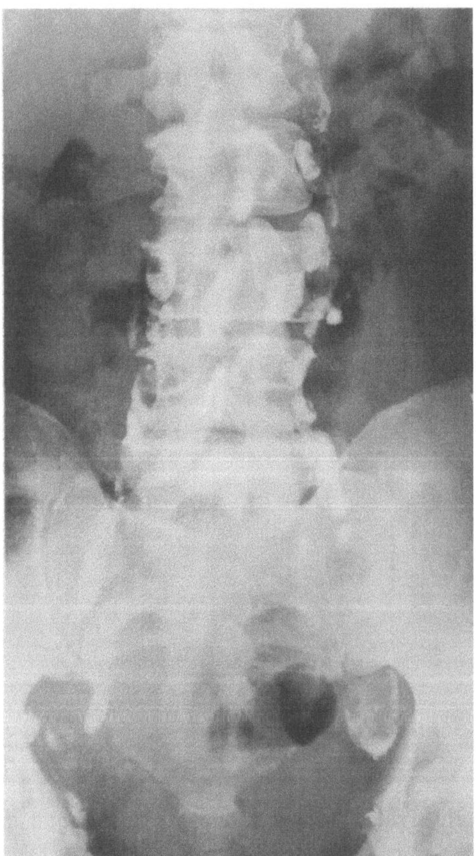

Fig. 5. At the time of lymphography a grossly involved node is seen on the left side of the pelvis and a smaller involved node is seen on the right. Nodes that maybe involved are seen in the para-aortic region

5 Incidence of Abnormal Lymphograms

The three criteria discussed above have been used to classify the results of lymphography in 74 patients with previously untreated carcinoma of the prostate (Table 1). There is an overall incidence of involved nodes in 51% of patients, and 25% of these had involved para-aortic nodes. In no case were abnormal para-aortic nodes found without involved nodes being seen in the pelvis. The patient with a T0 tumour and a positive lymphogram is interesting and merits further discussion. At prostatectomy for what was considered to be benign prostatic hyperplasia a small prostatic carcinoma was found. A lymphogram performed shortly afterwards showed highly suggestive nodes on the left side of the pelvis (Figs. 7 and 8). Following radiotherapy to the pelvis the appearances were as in Fig. 9. The nodes which were under suspicion before treatment had contracted by 38% compared with a selection of normal nodes in the pelvis, which had only contracted by 28%. The method used in this assessment has been described by McIvor et al. (1980), and according to our criteria these nodes must be considered to have been involved, because of their behaviour on follow-up films after radiotherapy.

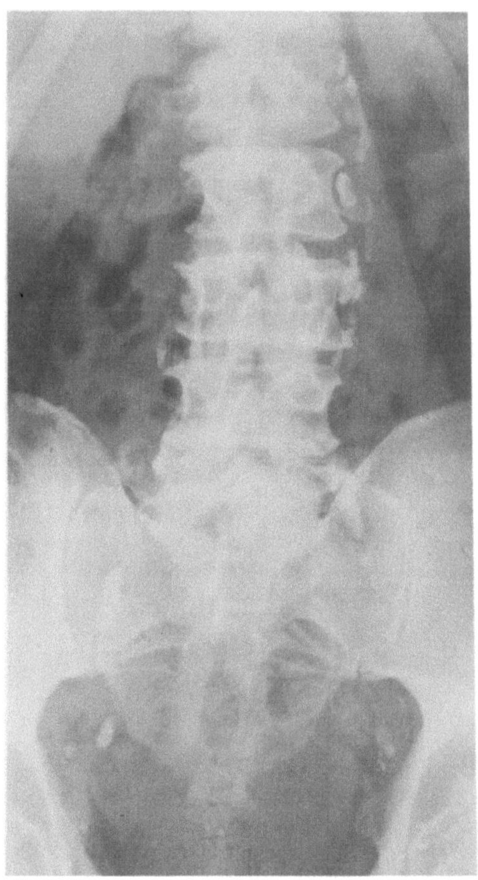

Fig. 6. Following radiotherapy there has been rapid reduction in the volume of the involved nodes, but no change in the doubtful nodes except loss of contrast medium. The para-aortic nodes have not behaved like involved nodes and therefore do not contain deposits

Table 1. Carcinoma of prostate: Extent of primary tumour and lymphogram result in 74 untreated patients

Primary tumour	Patients	Lymphogram positive	Lymphogram negative
T0	11	1 (9%)	10 (91%)
T1	10	3 (30%)	7 (70%)
T2	16	7 (44%)	9 (56%)
T3	18	11 (61%)	7 (39%)
T4	19	16 (84%)	3 (16%)
Total	74	38 (51%)	36 (49%)

There was no histological confirmation of these findings, since it is not the policy at the Royal Marsden Hospital to perform lymphadenectomies on patients with carcinoma of the prostate. According to the same diagnostic criteria in patients with carcinoma of the cervix managed by Wertheim's hysterectomy and lymphadenectomy, the accuracy of lymphography was of the order of 90%. It is also interesting to compare the figures in Table 1 with the results of a previously published smaller series of 45 new patients (Paxton et al. 1975); the rates of lymph node involvement by stage are reasonably consistent: T0, nil; T1, 25%; T2, 46%; T3, 60%; T4, 92%.

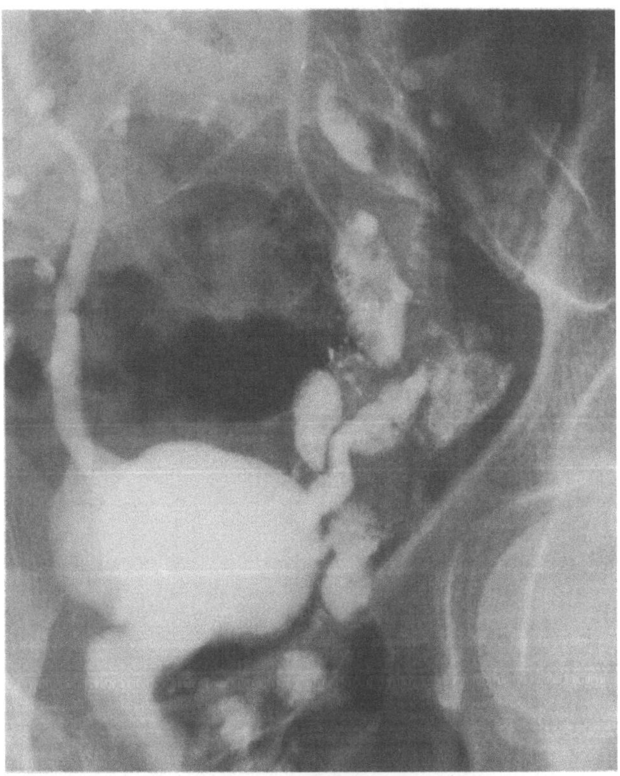

Fig. 7. Patient with carcinoma of the prostate, stage T0. Possibly positive nodes are seen in the left side of the pelvis on the oblique view

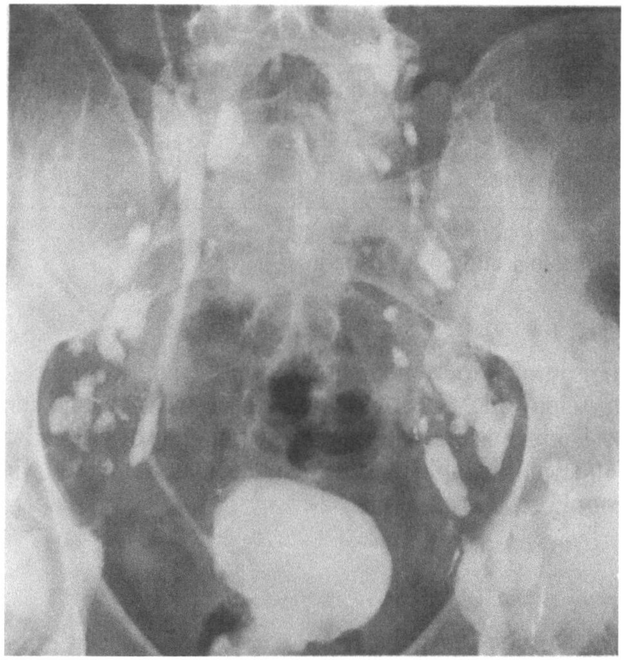

Fig. 8. Same patient as in Fig. 7. Lymphogram (*AP view*) shows suggestive nodes in the left side of the pelvis

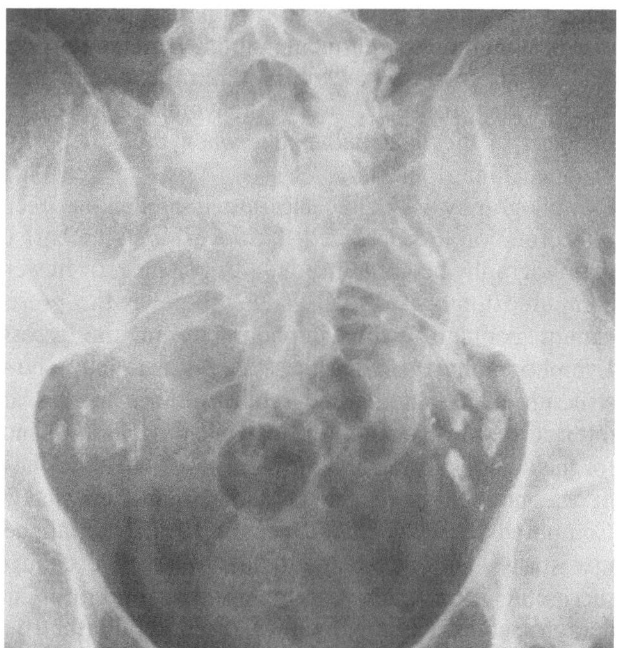

Fig. 9. Same patient as in Fig. 7. AP view following radiotherapy. The nodes considered possibly positive have contracted differentially compared with the normal nodes (38% as against 28%). These nodes are therefore considered to have contained metastases

Table 2. Carcinoma of prostate: positive lymph nodes

Study	No. of patients	T1 + T2	T3
Macdonald (present study)	74	38%	61%[a]
Hilaris et al. (1977)	208	29%	59%[b]
Spellman et al. (1977)	69	20%	64%[b]
O'Donoghue et al. (1976)	20	12%	44%[b]

[a] Lymphography only
[b] Histologically positives nodes

It is useful to compare this purely lymphographic series with other series where histology has been obtained either from lymphadenectomy (Hilaris et al. 1977; O'Donoghue et al. 1976) or from sampling of suggestive nodes (Spellman et al. 1977). The lymphographic series compares reasonably well with the two larger, histologically monitored series (Table 2).

6 Clinical Applications

The presence of lymph node metastases in patients with carcinoma of the prostate is an important factor in prognosis (Flocks 1973; Hilaris et al. 1977) and they may be demonstrated in the absence of other evidence of metastases. Radiotherapy is an effective method of treatment (Bloom and Hendry 1973; this volume, Chap. 10), but it is necessary to know how localised or otherwise the tumour is, and it is also important to know the precise location of the lymphatic nodes. Lymphography will demonstrate deposits in the opacified nodes when these deposits have grown large enough to produce filling defects.

Lymphography is highly accurate if meticulous techniques and strict criteria for interpretation are observed. However, a statement such as this is not enough. Has lymphography been superseded, for instance, by newer diagnostic techniques, such as computed tomography (CT)? In the pelvis the present generation of CT scanners cannot compete with lymphography in the assessment of the lateral nodes. Lymphography opacifies these nodes and may show alterations in their internal structure. Computed tomography outlines masses and does not at present show internal structure and therefore, while it is by far the most efficient technique available for the demonstration of large metastases when they have extended outside the capsule of the node it is unable to show small deposits within the normal-sized node. Computed tomography is also unable to differentiate between an enlarged node due to metastasis and one enlarged due to reactive changes. As yet CT has not been successful in assessing accurately the obturator nodes that are normally not demonstrated by lymphography. In an unpublished series comparing lymphography and CT in the assessment of pelvic nodes in 95 patients with pelvic tumours there was a discrepancy in the findings in 25 patients (Hodson, unpublished work). In 24 of these patients lymphography was considered to be correct, and CT in one. Most of the problems occurred in patients with deposits in normal-sized nodes. In the para-aortic region, however, CT is much more sensitive and can almost always be used in those patients in whom lymphography fails or is considered to be unsuitable.

In carcinoma of the prostate, lymphography, despite its limitations, seems to give valuable information to be used in planning treatment for individual patients, particularly for those with no other evidence of distant metastases.

7 References

Bloom HJG, Hendry WF (1973) Treatment of prostatic cancer. In: Raven RW (ed) Modern trends in oncology, vol 1, Part 2. Butterworths, London, p 143

Flocks RH (1973) The treatment of stage C prostatic cancer with special reference to combined surgical and radiation therapy. J Urol 109: 462–463

Flocks RH, Culp D, Porto R (1959) Lymphatic spread from prostatic cancer. J Urol 81: 194–196

Hilaris BS, Whitmore WF, Batata M, Barzell W (1977) Behavioral patterns of prostate adenocarcinoma following an ^{125}I implant and pelvic node dissection. Int J Radiat Oncol Biol Phys 2: 631–637

Macdonald JS (1976) In: Ansell G (ed) Complications in diagnostic radiology. Blackwell Scientific Publications, Oxford, pp 301–316

McIvor J, Massouh H, Backhouse BM, MacRae KD (1980) Lymphography in prostatic carcinoma – Implications for the diagnosis of metastases. Br J Radiol 53: 74–80

O'Donoghue EPN, Shiridhar P, Sherwood T, Williams JP, Chisholm GD (1976) Lymphography and pelvic lymphadenectomy in carcinoma of the prostate. Br J Urol 48: 689–696

Paxton RM, Williams G, Macdonald JS (1975) Role of lymphography in carcinoma of the prostate. Br Med J i: 120–122

Spellman MC, Castellino RA, Ray GR, Pistenma DA, Bagshaw MA (1977) An evaluation of lymphography in localised carcinoma of the prostate. Radiology 125: 637–644

Nuclear Medicine

M. V. Merrick, A. R. Stone, and G. D. Chisholm

Departments of Nuclear Medicine and Urology, Western General Hospital,
GB – Edinburgh

1 Introduction

The major application of nuclear medicine in the diagnosis and management of cancer of the prostate is undoubtedly the detection of skeletal metastases. A number of attempts have been made to image the primary tumour itself, to image metastases, and to detect lymph node involvement. None of these, however, has yet been successful.

2 Imaging of Primary Carcinoma

Three approaches have been employed in the imaging of primaries in the prostate. Non-specific cancer-seeking agents such as gallium and indium bleomycin have been used, but the large amount of excreted activity present in the bladder and rectum would preclude identification of the prostate even if there was significant uptake within it.

The prostate, like the pancreas, contains relatively high concentrations of zinc. In both organs zinc is present as a complex metalloprotein which is stable and has a long turnover time compared with the half-time of simple zinc salts in plasma. The incorporation of inorganic zinc into either the prostate or tumours of that organ is, not surprisingly, insufficient for imaging to be possible (Chisholm et al. 1974).

The third approach has been the use of labelled oestrogens. There is evidence that oestrogen receptors exist in the prostate. It is possible to iodinate the steroid nucleus in one of a number of positions. There is no useful concentration of iodinated steroid analogues in the prostate, however, either in experimental animals or in man. There are good theoretical reasons for doubting that this approach is likely to be profitable. Firstly, the mechanisms in vivo for deiodination of the steroid nucleus are very efficient, and it is unlikely that any iodinated steroids will survive for long. Secondly, the technique is based on the assumption that steroids are bound to specific receptor sites in the prostate more strongly than they are to non-specific sites. There is no evidence that this is true. Thirdly, there are in any case relatively few specific receptors compared with the large number of non-specific sites. To obtain preferential binding to specific sites it would be necessary to administer the labelled steroid at a specific

Recent Results in Cancer Research, Vol. 78
© Springer-Verlag Berlin · Heidelberg 1981

activity at least 100 times greater than it has yet been possible to synthesise (Eckelman et al. 1978).

A fourth approach has been employed with some tumours, although not carcinoma of the prostate, namely the use of labelled antibodies (Dykes et al. 1980). Uptake has only been reported in very large tumours readily detectable by conventional techniques. Indeed the problem with all attempts at direct imaging of tumours in vivo is the very high tumour-to-background ratio which would be necessary for there to be any hope of visualising tumours not readily detectable by clinical examination of simple radiological techniques. The actual ratio required is in excess of 100 : 1. If such a substance were to be found it would clearly have important therapeutic applications. Unfortunately such a compound is likely to remain within the realms of science fiction.

3 Lymph Node Visualisation

The primary drainage of the prostate is via the internal iliac lymph nodes, which are not accessible to conventional techniques of radiological lymphography. No lymphatics have been identified within the gland itself, although the capsule is well supplied (Smith 1966; Shridhar 1979).

Radioisotope imaging of lymph nodes, or lymphoscintigraphy, has been used for over 20 years, particularly on the continent of Europe, but has never achieved much popularity in the English-speaking world. Recently there has been an upsurge of interest in its use, particularly in the detection of the internal mammary nodes, and it has recently been shown to be a reliable technique of staging carcinoma of the breast (Black et al. 1980). A number of workers, including ourselves, have looked at it as a means of imaging internal iliac nodes, but to date the results have been disappointing (Gardiner et al. 1979; Stone et al. 1979).

It is sometimes possible to visualise internal iliac nodes, but it cannot be done consistently. It is not to be expected that filling defects will be identified within nodes, but judging by experience at other sites there should be non-filling of nodes containing even very small amounts of tumour. However, to use non-filling as a diagnostic criterion it is first necessary to have a technique which gives reliable visualisation of the normal node. A number of possible sites of injection have been investigated but none has been found which gives consistent visualisation. The reason for this is not altogether clear. It is thought, although there is no conclusive evidence, that the site of injection may be crucial.

By analogy with experience in the breast, where reliable visualisation of the axillary nodes can be achieved by an intradermal injection, but not following subcutaneous injection, it is reasonable to postulate that the site of injection is the limiting factor. If, as appears to be the case, the lymphatic plexus within the prostate is negligible or non-existent, and the only well-developed plexus is that in the capsule, it may be that the target into which the colloid must be injected, namely the capsule, is so thin that it cannot be hit with sufficient reliability. Alternative sites of injection, such as the mucosa of the rectum, do not appear to yield reproducible results, nor are they attractive, because of the risk of infection. Thus at the moment visualisation of the internal iliac nodes cannot be achieved with any clinically useful degree of reproducibility.

4 Skeletal Metastases – Bone Scanning

The incidence of skeletal metastases at autopsy in patients with carcinoma of the prostate has been reported as between 50% and 70%, similar to that found in carcinoma of the breast and Hodgkin's disease (McNeil 1978). The incidence of abnormal bone scans at presentation is lower than this, being variously reported as between 20% and 50% (Merrick 1975; O'Donoghue et al. 1978).
The mechanism of incorporation of all imaging agents into the skeleton is probably similar. Tracer passes from the blood into the extravascular water by passive diffusion. There is a certain amount of exchange between the extracellular fluid and the surface layers of the bone mineral crystal. This occurs in all parts of the body, but is a comparatively slow process. Where mineral is being formed its ionic composition represents the composition of the extracellular fluid at that point. Therefore the addition of a tracer to the extracellular fluid where bone is being formed results in the incorporation of that tracer into the bone mineral.
The extraction ratio (i.e., the percentage of the activity in the arterial blood that is removed on a single passage through an organ) for the older bone scanning agents such as fluorine and strontium is high, at least 80%, and possibly close to 100% in the case of fluorine. The extraction ratio for all the technetium agents is much lower, between 25% and 40% (Merrick and Smith 1980). Theoretically, agents with a high extraction ratio should show a greater difference between normal and abnormal tissue, but in practice, if this occurs, the difference is too small to be clinically relevant.

4.1 Agents

The commonest bone scanning agents in current use are technetium pyrophosphate (TcPYP), technetium ethanehydroxydiphosphonate (TcEHDP), and technetium methylenediphosphate (TcMDP). TcMDP is the most widely used at present, because its rate of clearance from the blood is faster than that of any of the others. Some workers have observed a higher lesion-to-normal bone ratio with TcEHDP than with the other technetium agents (Fogleman et al. 1979). However, the experience of other workers suggests that any difference in this ratio is too small to be clinically significant (Rudd et al. 1977; Rosenthall et al. 1977), and the faster and more reliable blood clearance of TcMDP at least off-sets any such difference.
Thus the bone scan represents the rate of new bone formation, whereas the X-ray shows the total mineral content. The presence of a metastasis may produce both bone destruction (by stimulating osteoclastic activity) and repair or osteoblastic activity. An abnormality is visible on a plain radiograph only when there is a large net imbalance between the competing processes. The scan and the radiograph are not related in any simple manner; indeed under many circumstances there may be an inverse relationship – as blood flow and turnover decrease, the mineral content increases. The extreme example of this may be found in conditions such as osteopetrosis, where the dense bones are for all practical purposes dead and there is neither blood flow through them nor uptake of bone scanning agents into them.
The criteria of a technically adequate bone scan are that a sufficient number of counts shall have been collected to distinguish between random statistical noise and true differences in count rate in adjacent areas, and secondly that the clearance of activity

from soft tissues is sufficient for small differences in count rate between adjacent parts of the skeleton not to be obscured. Lesions will undoubtedly be missed if the scans are performed too soon after injection or too rapidly, or if insufficient isotope is administered.

4.2 Imaging Equipment

The choice of equipment is to some extent dictated by what is available. The old-fashioned rectilinear scanner should not be spurned, although it is rather restricted in its speed. Because of the comparatively small detector area, and hence the low sensitivity, it is necessary to use relatively low-resolution collimators if adequate statistics are to be collected, but nevertheless good results can be obtained with these instruments if sufficient time and care are taken.

The majority of centres today use a gamma camera, either a static large-field camera or a scanning camera, principally because it is the most versatile instrument for the whole range of investigations performed. Few departments can afford a dedicated instrument for one examination only. It is not generally appreciated that conversion of a static gamma camera into a moving (scanning) camera involves a significant loss of resolution. As little or no time is saved by scanning instead of taking the eight or so views necessary to cover the whole body with a large-field camera, there seems little point, other than aesthetics, in using this attachment. The major drawback with the gamma camera is the extreme dependence of resolution on distance from the collimator face, the resolution falling off very rapidly indeed. The gamma camera is therefore a very good machine for detecting lesions in the rib or spinous process, but is relatively poor for detecting lesions in the pelvis or vertebral bodies. Moreover, when it is used as a static instrument it is possible to position the patient in contact with the machine, while when it is used as a scanning camera the patient has to be separated from the machine, thereby further impairing the resolution of the scanning system.

The alternative instrument is the multi-detector scanner. This is in effect a 20-hcaded scanner and, because of the much larger surface area of the detectors, permits high-resolution collimators to be employed. This machine has the advantage that the collimators are not only of higher resolution, but also of a long focal length, and the resolution is much less dependent on depth. The chances of detecting a lesion are therefore almost as high for one situated deeply as one near the surface. Although there are no systematic studies comparing the three types of instruments there are some preliminary data which suggest that the pick-up rate of lesions with the multi-detector scanner is higher than that with the gamma camera.

4.3 Accuracy

There has been a good deal of argument as to whether the bone scan should be performed before or after the radiological skeletal survery. To some extent, in the case of carcinoma of the prostate, this question is academic, as the majority of prostatic carcinomas are diagnosed after the patient has been investigated for benign prostatic hyperplasia and therefore has already had chest X-rays and excretion urography. In the patient who has had no recent X-rays, the bone scan is the initial examination of choice, as there is now ample evidence that it will reveal more metastatic cases and significantly more lesions than the radiological skeletal survey (Buck et al. 1975; O'Donoghue et al. 1978). If the bone scan is abnormal it is necessary to take X-rays of at least some of the areas. Once the presence of one metastasis has been confirmed it is to some extent academic to prove that every lesion is metastatic.

The bone scan is an examination with a very high sensitivity but a very low specificity. The demonstration of an abnormality on the scan is not synonymous with the presence of metastatic disease. The sensitivity of the bone scan in carcinoma of the prostate is higher than in other malignancies. False-negatives have been reported in older series, in which the radiopharmaceutical employed was strontium 85 or strontium 87m, but have not been reported when technically adequate scans were obtained with fluorine 18 or the technetium radiopharmaceuticals. However, degenerative joint disease, infection, osteomalacia, Paget's disease, and various other conditions can give rise to focal abnormalities on the scan, which can therefore be interpreted only in conjunction with contemporary radiographs of the appropriate regions. Many of the conditions listed can readily be diagnosed on plain films, and in other cases there is unequivocal radiological evidence of metastatic disease. In some cases equivocal radiological appearances can be confidently interpreted as either normal or abnormal if the radiographic and scan appearances are considered together.

There remain a number of lesions where there is a definite abnormality on the scan, but normal radiographs. Further radiographic views and tomograms will sometimes clarify the position, but in a few cases a definitive diagnosis can be obtained only by biopsy or follow-up. If the scan is normal it is still necessary to take at least one X-ray picture, preferably of the chest, as disseminated disease can sometimes be so symmetrical as to mimic a normal scan (Osmond et al. 1975). The features which should give rise to the suspicion of this phenomenon are the presence of a very high-quality bone scan with very little soft-tissue background, little or no renal activity, and an unusually clearly defined skeleton. Some workers have reported a high incidence of false-negative bone scans in the pelvis (Galasko and Doyle 1972). These are for the most part earlier papers describing studies in which old, comparatively low-resolution gamma cameras were used. In our experience there is no difficulty in diagnosing metastases in the pelvis provided that the patient has been able to empty the bladder. However, in patients with a large residual volume an X-ray examination of the pelvis is advisable.

Lesions may occur in any bone, but the vast majority occur in the axial skeleton. Shirazi et al. (1974) reported a series of 1,265 bone scans, 112 of which were performed in in-patients with carcinoma of the prostate. In only five of these 112 was there a solitary lesion. Extremities were involved in 27. Solitary lesions in the extremity are very rare indeed, and if time is limited it may be justifiable to discontinue the scan after the axial skeleton has been examined, and not examine the legs. Particular caution must be exercised when a solitary rib lesion, or lesions in adjacent ribs are present, as these are commonly due to trivial trauma not producing any radiological abnormality.

4.4 Incidence of Abnormal Scans

Of more importance than the overall gross yield of abnormal bone scans is the distribution of abnormality by T stage (Table 1). Buck et al. (1975) reported abnormal scans in four of 20 T0 patients, but did not specify the incidence in more advanced stages. O'Donoghue et al. (1978) found two abnormal scans in ten patients with T0 tumours, while Schaefer, quoted by McNeil (1978), gives a yield of 7% abnormal studies in stage T1 and stage T2. In our present series abnormal scans were found in eight of 24 patients with T0 disease. There is a striking difference between the findings in cancer of the prostate and those in breast carcinoma, where the majority of studies now reveal the incidence of abnormal scans in patients with T0 disease to be under 5%. As can be seen from Table 1, the incidence increases as the T category increases, reaching 69% in patients with T4 disease, not significantly different from the incidence at post-mortem. The comparative rarity of T1 tumours in all series, and the low incidence of abnormal bone scans in them, raises the possibility that these may be in some way different from other prostatic carcinomas.

The relationship between T and M staging is shown in Table 2. Of the 25 patients who presented with stage T0 or T1, 16 had M0 and nine had M1 disease. However, of the 75 patients with T2–4 tumours, 50 had evidence of metastatic disease. Not surprisingly, the majority of T0 and T1 tumours were graded histologically as well-differentiated cancers (Table 3) whereas many more of the T2–4 tumours were moderately or poorly differentiated. What is perhaps more surprising is the lack of correlation between M staging at presentation and histological differentiation. As can be seen from Table 3 there is no correlation between these parameters.

The incidence of abnormal bone scans in the present series is somewhat higher than in most of those previously reported. Abnormal scans were found in 54 of 100 patients; the X-ray appearances were also abnormal in 40. Thus there were 14 patients who at presentation had abnormal scans but no radiographic evidence of metastatic disease, giving a sensitivity of 1.0 for the bone scan and 0.74 for routine radiology.

There were 59 patients who were staged M1 at presentation, and 54 of these had an abnormal bone scan (Table 5). In the remainder the evidence was based on a raised acid phosphatase. The significance of this may be questioned. There was no patient with other evidence of dissemination who did not also have an abnormal scan. It is therefore clear that the bone scan is by far the most sensitive indicator of dissemination in this disease. The only other test for which a similar sensitivity has been claimed is 24-h urinary hydroxyproline excretion (Bichler et al. 1978). In view of the variation of the normal range with age, nutritional status, and therapy, however, further experience is necessary before their conclusions can be accepted. The sensitivity of both acid and alkaline phosphatase is much lower, and both suffer from both false-positive and false-negative findings (Shafer and Reinke 1977).

4.5 Assessment of Response

There is now general agreement that the bone scan is by far the most sensitive single test of metastases in patients with carcinoma of the prostate. There is less general agreement on its value in follow-up. As with carcinoma of the breast, a significant minority of patients who are initially scan-negative will develop abnormal scans on follow-up. In our previous study (Buck et al. 1977) two of 33 patients without initial evidence of skeletal metastases developed evidence of metastatic disease, i.e., an abnormal bone scan, during follow-up of between 2 and 5 years. Fitzpatrick et al. (1978) found a higher conversion rate, 19 of 99. In our present series the change from a normal to an abnormal scan, or an increase in the number of lesions visible compared with a previous abnormal scan (Fig. 1) occurred in 22 of the 24 patients in whom there

Table 1a. Incidence of abnormal bone scan by T stage

	T0		T1		T2	
	Total	Abnormal	Total	Abnormal	Total	Abnormal
Buck et al. (1975)	20	4	5	0	–	–
O'Donoghue et al. (1978)	10	2	3	0	15	0
Present authors	24	8	1	0	14	6
Overall	54	14 (26%)	9	0		

Table 1b

	T3		T4	
	Total	Abnormal	Total	Abnormal
Buck et al. (1975)	–	–	–	–
O'Donoghue et al. (1978)	48	24	14	8
Present authors	49	29	12	10
Overall	97	53 (55%)	26	18 (69%)

–, Not stated

Table 2. Relationship between T and M stages

	T stage		Total
	T0–1	T2–4	
M stage			
M0	16	25	41
M1	9	50	59
Total	25	75	100

Table 3. Relationship between T stage and histological grading

Stage at presentation	Histological grade				
	Well-differentiated	Moderately differentiated	Poorly differentiated	Not known	Total
T0–1	17	3	0	5	25
T2–4	27	15	16	17	75
Total	44	18	16	22	100

Table 4. Relationship between M stage and histological grading

Stage at presentation	Histological grade				
	Well-differentiated	Moderately differentiated	Poorly differentiated	Not known	Total
M0	20	9	8	4	41
M1	24	9	8	18	59
Total	44	18	16	22	100

Table 5. Evidence of metastatic disease (M1)

Acid phosphatase only	5
Bone scan + X-ray	8
Bone scan only	10
Bone scan + acid phosphatase	4
Bone scan + X-ray + acid phosphatase	32

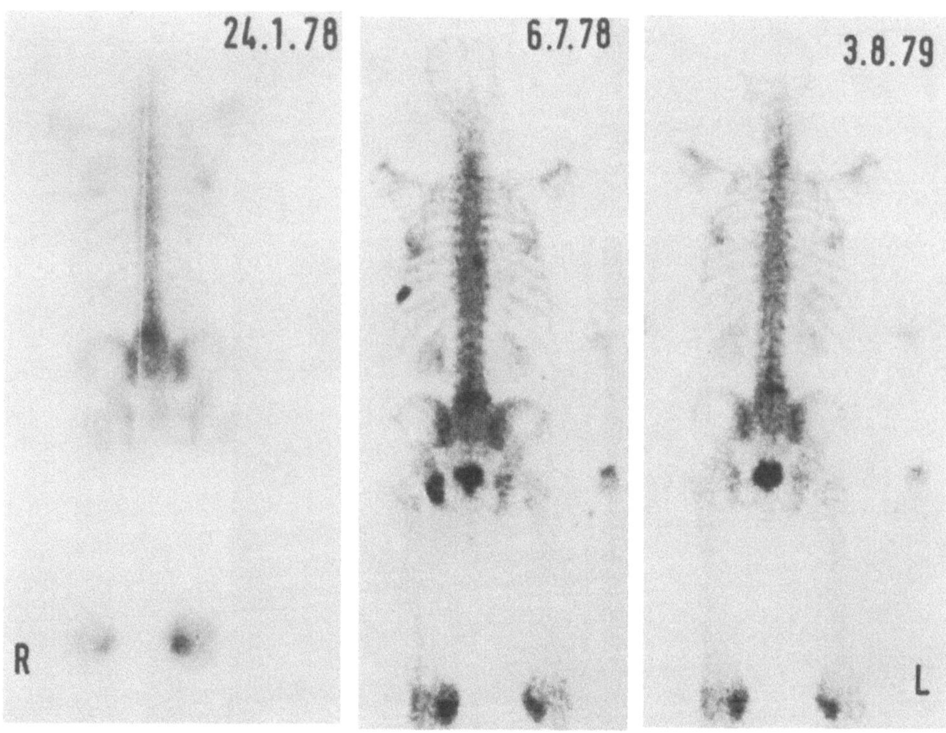

Fig. 1. Scan on 24. 1. 78 shows increased uptake in L4/5 owing to spondylosis, otherwise normal. By 6. 7. 78 lesions are visible in the right 8th rib, D7, and the right ischium. Stilboestrol medication was started. By 3. 8. 79 the lesion in D7 has disappeared and the others are barely visible

was objective evidence of progression of the disease. The scan preceded other evidence of deterioration in nine of these patients, and was the sole evidence of deterioration in two.

During the period of follow-up 19 patients died. Only two of the deaths were amongst the 47 patients who had a normal bone scan at the time of diagnosis, a mortality of 4%. In contrast, there were 17 deaths amongst the 53 patients with abnormal scans, a mortality of 32%. An abnormal scan therefore clearly carries a much poorer prognosis.

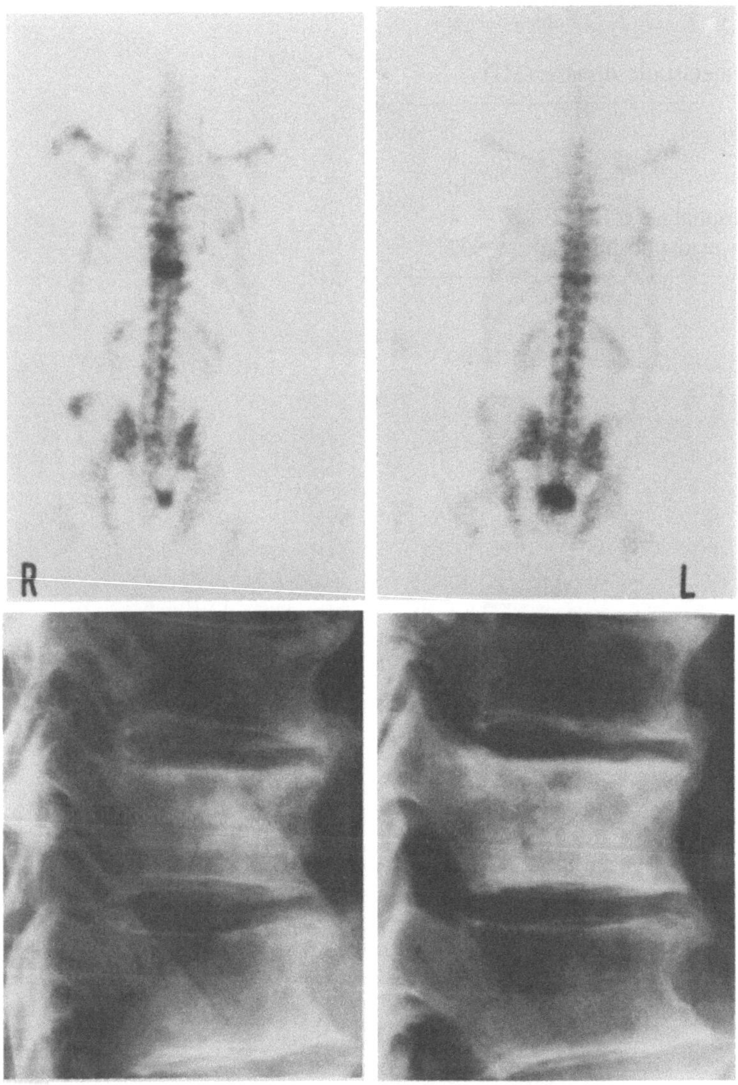

Fig. 2. Initial scan shows increased uptake in *left* 5th rib, D7, D9, and the *right* ileum. One year later, after stilboestrol medication only the lesion in D9 and the ileum remain visible. Radiographs show that there has been a considerable increase of sclerosis in D9 between the two scans. The reduced count rate is partly due to reduced osteoblastic activity, but partly also to the increased bone density, acting as a filter

It is more difficult to decide how to evaluate clinical improvement on the scan. A reduction in count rate compared with the previous examination may indicate healing, but is commonly associated with increasing sclerosis (Fig. 2). There is significant attenuation of the 140 keV gamma photons of technetium by bone, and any increase in bone density will be associated with increased attenuation and therefore fewer detected photons. As the isotope is distributed in a non-uniform manner in an inhomogeneous absorbing medium it is not possible to correct this attenuation accurately. It is therefore impossible to state in any given case to what extent a reduction in detected activity represents a true reduction in osteoblastic function, and to what extent it represents increased bone density.

A further objection to the use of the bone scan other than as a crude assessment of response is the fact that it is not a direct indicator of tumour activity, but rather of response to the tumour. It is conceivable, indeed probable, that tumour regression may, at least initially, be associated with increased osteoblastic activity as repair proceeds apace.

Attempts to 'quantitate' response to treatment from the bone scan are therefore unlikely to have any advantages over simple numeration. Even this is fraught with difficulty, as it is not uncommon to find some lesions regressing and other new ones becoming apparent simultaneously.

In summary, the bone scan remains the most valuable single test in staging of carcinoma of the prostate, and has an important role during follow-up.

References

Bichler KH, Harzmann R, Heller W, et al. (1978) Bony metastases from cancer of the prostate. Aktuelle Urologie 9:21–28

Black RB, Merrick MV, Taylor TV, Forrest APM (1980) Staging of carcinoma of the breast by lymphoscintigraphy. Lancet 2:15–17

Buck AC, Chisholm GD, Merrick MV, Lavender JP (1975) Br J Urol 47:287–294

Buck AC, Chisholm GD, Merrick MV (1977) Follow-up of prostate carcinoma with serial bone scanning using cyclotron-produced 18-fluorine. Recent Results Cancer Res 60:81–96

Chisholm GD, Short MD, Ghanadian R, McRae CU, Glass HI (1974) Radiozinc uptake and scintiscanning in prostatic disease. J Nucl Med 15:739–742

Dykes PW, Hine KR, Bradwell AR, Blackburn JC, Reeder TA, Drolc Z, Booth SN (1980) Localisation of tumour deposits by external scanning after injection of radiolabelled anti carcinoembryonic antigen. Br Med J 280:220–222

Eckelman WC, Reba RC (1978) Classification of radiotracers. J Nucl Med 19:79–81

Fitzpatrick JM, Constable AR, Sherwood T, Shephenson JJ, et al. (1978) Serial bone scanning: the assessment of treatment response in carcinoma of the prostate. Br J Urol 50:555–561

Fogelman I, Citrin DC, McKillop JH, Turner JE, Bessent RG, Greig WR (1979) A clinical comparison of Tc99m HEDP and Tc99m MDP in the detection of bone metastases. J Nucl Med 20:98–101

Galasko CSB, Doyle FH (1972) The detection of skeletal metastases from mammary cancer. A regional comparison between radiology and scintigraphy. Clin Radiol 23:295–297

Gardiner RA, Fitzpatrick JM, Constable AR, Cranage RW, et al. (1979) Improved techniques in radionuclide imaging of prostatic lymph nodes. Br J Urol 51:561–564

McNeil BJ (1978) Rationale for the use of bone scans in selected metastatic and primary bone tumours. Semin Nucl Med 8:336–345

Merrick MV (1975) Bone scanning. Br J Radiol 48: 327–351 (review article)
Merrick MV, Smith MA (1980) Radioisotope investigation of the skeleton. In: Goodfellow J, Owen H (eds) Scientific foundations of orthopaedics. Heinemann, London, pp 342–356
O'Donoghue EPN, Constable AR, Sherwood T, Stevenson JJ, Chisholm GD (1978) Bone scanning and plasma phosphatases in carcinoma of the prostate. Br J Urol 50: 172–188
Osmond JD, Pendergrass HP, Potsaid MJ (1975) Accuracy of 99mTc diphosphonate bone scans and roentgenograms in the detection of prostate, breast and lung carcinoma metastases. Am J Roentgenol 125: 972–977
Rosenthall L, Arzoumanian A, Lisbona R, Itch K (1977) A longitudinal comparison of the kinetics of 99mTcMDP and 99mTcEHDP in humans, Clin Nucl Med 2: 232–234
Rudd TG, Allen DR, Hartnett DE (1977) Tc-99m methylene diphosphonate versus Tc-99m pyrophosphate: biologic and clinical comparison. J Nucl Med 18: 872–876
Shafer RB, Reinke DB (1977) Contribution of bone scan, serum acid and alkaline phosphatase and radiographic bone survey to the management of newly diagnosed carcinoma of the prostate. Clin Nucl Med 2: 200–203
Shirazi PH, Rayudu GVS, Fordham EW (1974) 18F Bone scanning: Review of indications and results of 1500 scans. Radiology 112: 361–368
Shridhar P (1979) The lymphatics of the prostate gland and their role in the spread of prostatic carcinoma. Ann R Coll Surg Engl 61: 115–122
Smith MJV (1966) The lymphatics of the prostate. Invest Urol 3: 439–444
Stone AR, Merrick MV, Chisholm GD (1979) Prostatic lymphoscintigraphy. Br J Urol 51: 556–560

Surgery

W. F. Hendry

St. Bartholomews and Royal Marsden Hospital, Institute of Urology, GB – London

1 Introduction

The surgeon's first responsibility in the management of carcinoma of the prostate is to detect the presence of the disease. Malignancy may be suspected on digital palpation of the prostate, and then microscopic evidence must be provided by biopsy. Alternatively, the carcinoma may be discovered incidentally in tissue removed for the correction of bladder-neck obstruction. Whichever way the tumour is diagnosed, it is the surgeon's next responsibility to define the stage of the disease – the local extent of the primary growth, whether it is necessary to study the pelvic lymph nodes, and whether there is any evidence of distant metastases. More difficult, an attempt should be made to gauge the malignant potential of the tumour in a particular patient. Once this information is assembled, the surgeon has to choose the best therapeutic approach. He can try to cut out the cancer: but few of us believe that this is a valid first-line approach, especially with prostate carcinoma. If the patient is fortunate he may be entered into a well-thought-out, carefully constructed prospective trial. This will ensure that his disease is adequately staged, and management will be by one of two or more options which are appropriate for his disease at his age. In may be pointed out that there is evidence that patients in trials do better than those who are not (Lennox et al. 1979). The surgeon's contribution to the endocrine management of the patient may include orchidectomy and, later in the course of the disease, adrenalectomy or pituitary ablation.
In this presentation we shall consider the following aspects of the surgical management of prostatic cancer in turn: diagnosis, biopsy, staging, orchidectomy, and secondary endocrine therapy.

2 Diagnosis

How accurate is the surgeon's finger? Ten years ago, it was our practice to remove prostates that could be enucleated by retropubic prostatectomy, and far fewer transurethral resections (TURs) were performed. Before starting the prostatectomy, however, a very careful bimanual examination of the prostate was performed with the patient in the lithotomy position, to ensure that it could be enucleated; if there was any suspicion of malignancy, retropubic prostatectomy was avoided and in most cases a

Recent Results in Cancer Research, Vol. 78
© Springer-Verlag Berlin · Heidelberg 1981

Table 1. Correlation between digital assessment of the prostate under general anaesthesia and histological grade in 93 cases of prostatic cancer

Number of patients	Digital assessment	Histological grade			
		Focal	Good	Moderate	Poor
10	Benign	2	6	2	0
7	Firm, benign	1	4	1	1
25	Suggestive	0	1	8	6
61	Obvious Ca	0	6	24	31

needle biopsy was taken. Analysis of 94 patients with carcinoma of the prostate seen at St. Mary's General Hospital, Portsmouth in 1968/1970 showed that the diagnosis was missed completely in only ten patients (10.5%), and that in eight of these patients the disease was focal or well differentiated (Table 1). The prostate was noted to be firm but probably benign in a further seven patients; to arouse suspicion in 25; and to be obviously malignant in 61. The histological grade of malignancy became progressively worse as the diagnosis became more obvious. In 27 patients the disease was not diagnosed by needle biopsy. In 11 patients with prostates that felt benign or 'firm but probably benign', retropubic prostatectomy was performed. In a further 16 patients in whom transurethral prostatectomy had been performed, however, ten had prostates that aroused suspicion or were malignant. It is acknowledged that TUR is applicable to all prostates, irrespective of whether they can be enucleated or not, whereas to attempt to enucleate a prostate that is malignant is to invite complications.

There has been a swing towards transurethral prostatectomy in recent years, and few prostates are now enucleated. This has brought considerable benefits to the patient with bladder-neck obstruction, including shorter time in hospital, lower morbidity, and significantly reduced mortality (Chilton et al. 1978). The wider application of the transurethral operation to prostates irrespective of whether they are firm and even if they have a hard area, may have led to a less critical examination of prostates before surgery. Indeed, once the patient is draped and cysto-urethroscopy has been completed, it is common practice to proceed with resection of the prostate without risking contamination of the sterile area by repeating a rectal examination under anaesthetic. It follows that incidentally found carcinoma of the prostate (T0, see below) may be a much more heterogeneous group than the accurately defined discrete nodule (T1). Certainly the proportion of moderately or poorly differentiated tumours and the incidence of lymph node metastases were higher in the clinically undetected tumours, which showed diffuse infiltration of resected tissue compared with truly localised, early clinically detectable disease (Table 2; Golimbu and Morales 1979).

The trend towards greater use of transurethral prostatectomy may have led to reduced precision in the digital diagnosis of prostatic cancer, and as a result greater reliance may have to be placed on detailed examination of tissue removed by resection in defining the local extent of the disease (O'Donoghue and Pugh 1977), and on imaging techniques such as ultrasound (Peeling et al. 1979).

If the prostate arouses the suspicion of malignancy on digital examination, the surgeon must choose the best way to obtain tissue to establish the diagnosis. Although a full transurethral prostatectomy will nearly always confirm the diagnosis (Denton et al.

Table 2. Comparison of clinically undetected and detected early prostatic carcinomas. Golimbu and Morales (1979)

	A2 (T0; Diffuse)	Clinical stage	
		B1 (T1)	B2 (T2)
Well differentiated	21/94 (22%)	120/140 (86%)	10/25 (40%)
Moderately and poorly differentiated	75/94 (78%)	20/140 (14%)	15/25 (60%)
Lymph node metastases	12/53 (24%)	14/ 96 (14%)	34/86 (40%)

1967), there is good evidence that a needle biopsy is more reliable than a limited transurethral biopsy (Purser et al. 1967). A perineal or a transrectal approach may be used to obtain a needle biopsy: the rectal approach provides more direct access to the prostate and causes minimal morbidity (Daves et al. 1961), although antibiotic cover is advisable for a few days. The fine-needle aspiration technique (Franzén et al. 1960) causes minimal discomfort, and can be used in out-patients without anaesthesia (Fig. 1). The accuracy of the interpretation of the cytological smears, however, is dependent on the availability of a skilled cytologist. Provision of a core of prostatic tissue suitable for histological examination, for example by a Tru-Cut needle, requires a general anaesthetic. The Tru-Cut needle technique is more accurate for a reliable diagnosis was obtained in 95% of 80 patients, compared with only 82% of 138 patients with the Franzén technique (Hendry and Williams 1971). The fine-needle technique is undoubtedly useful in the conscious patient – e.g., in an out-patients' department – but if the results are unsatisfactory or unexpectedly negative, or if the patient requires a general anaesthetic, then a needle such as the Tru-Cut should be used to provide tissue for a histological diagnosis.

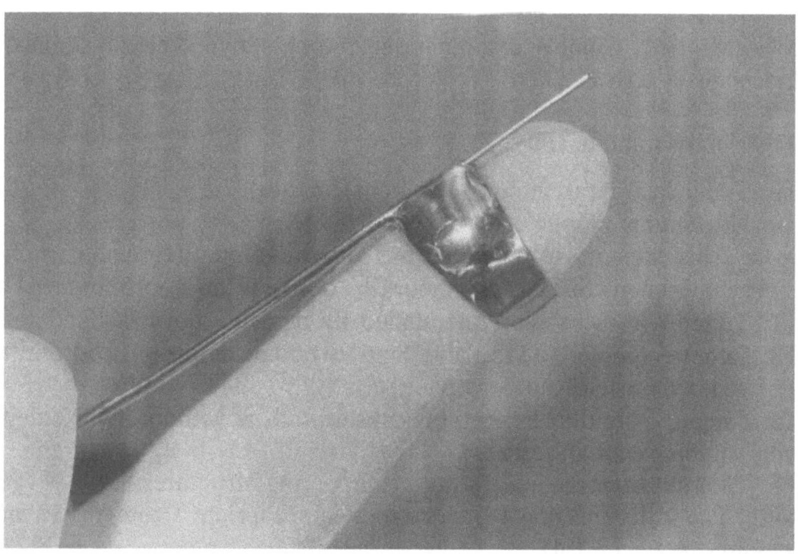

Fig. 1. The Franzén needle slips over the index finger and is suitable for prostatic biopsy without anaesthetic in out-patients

3 Staging

Many different systems of staging have been suggested by various groups interested in prostatic cancer. Unfortunately, their differences have made accurate international comparison of results impossible, and to overcome this the TNM system of tumour classification was introduced by the International Union against Cancer (UICC). The first classification proposed for the prostate proved difficult to use in clinical practice, and was revised in 1978 by the International TNM Subcommittee of the UICC. It provides an accurate shorthand method of recording the clinical (T) or pathological (pT) extent of the disease in the prostate and the presence or absence of disease in nodes (N) and of distant metastases (M). The adoption of this system should facilitate international comparison of results and enable the clinician to choose treatment for his patients more logically. The classification should be made when the patient first presents,but certain well-defined minimum criteria in the patients' assessment must be fulfilled before the TNM categorisation is undertaken. If these are not met for any reason the symbol X is assigned to the category in question.

The TNM System of Classification (UICC 1978)

The UICC classification applies only to carcinoma. There should be histological verification of the disease to permit division of cases by histological type. Any unconfirmed cases must be reported separately.
The following are the minimum requirements for assessment of the T, N, and M categories. If these cannot be met, the symbols TX, NX, and MX will be used.

T categories: Clinical examination, urography, endoscopy, and biopsy (if indicated) prior to definitive treatment.
N categories: Clinical examination and radiography, including lymphography and urography.
M categories: Clinical examination, radiography, skeletal studies, and relevant biochemical tests.

T: Primary tumour (Fig. 2).

Tis: Pre-invasive carcinoma (carcinoma in situ).
T0: No tumour palpable.
Note: This category includes the incidental finding of carcinoma in an operative or biopsy specimen. Such cases should be assigned an appropriate pT category.
T1: Tumour intracapsular surrounded by palpably normal gland.
T2: Tumour confined to the gland. Smooth nodule deforming contour, but lateral sulci and seminal vesicles not involved.
T3: Tumour extending beyond the capsule with or without involvement of the lateral sulci and/or seminal vesicles.
T4: Tumour fixed or infiltrating neighbouring structures.
Note: The suffix (m) may be added to the appropriate T category to indicate multiple tumours, e.g., T2 (m).
TX: The minimum requirements for assessment of the primary tumour cannot be met.

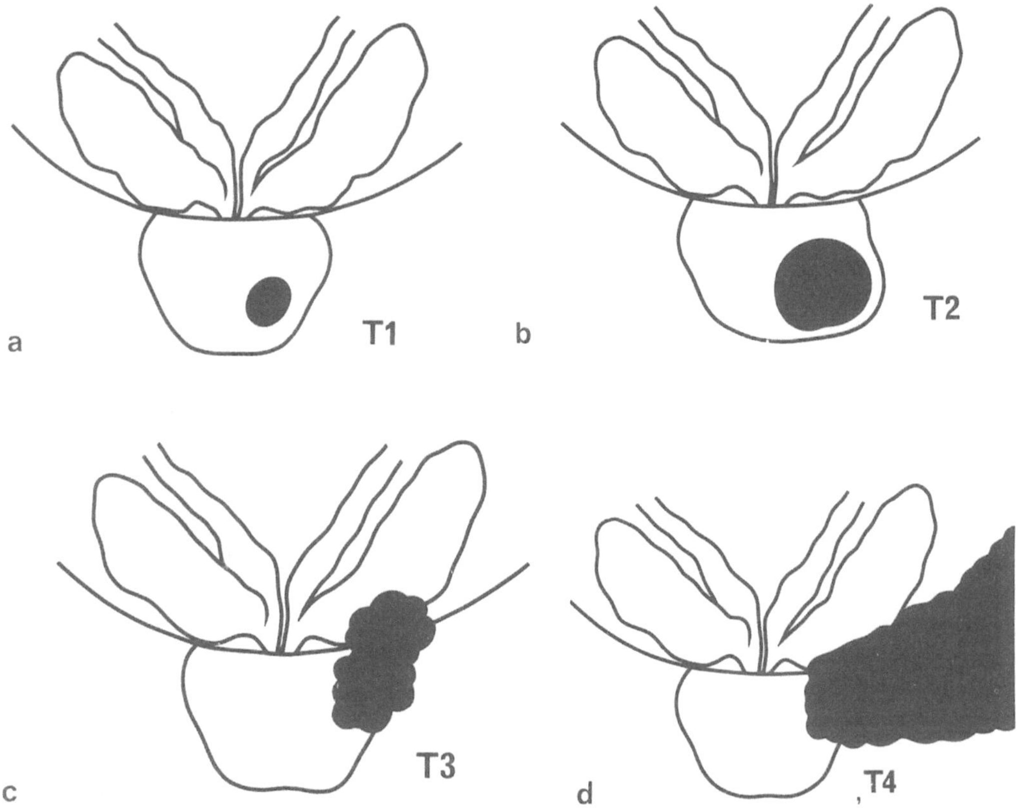

Fig. 2a–d. T classification for prostate: T0, incidental carcinoma; T1, intracapsular/normal gland (**a**); T2, intracapsular/deformed gland (**b**); T3, extension beyond capsule (**c**); T4, extension fixed to neighbouring organs (**d**) (See text for details)

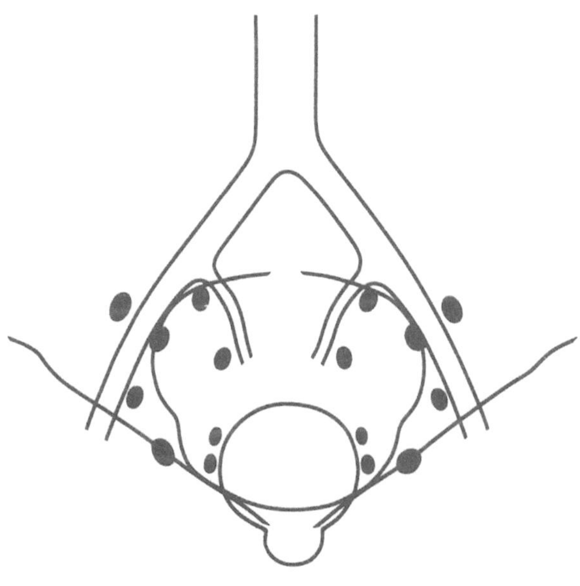

Fig. 3. Regional nodes for prostate. N1, single homolateral regional node; N2, contra- or bilateral/multiple regional nodes; N3, fixed regional nodes; N4, juxtaregional nodes (See text for details)

N: Regional and juxtaregional lymph nodes (Fig. 3).

The regional lymph nodes are the pelvic nodes below the bifurcation of the common iliac arteries; the juxtaregional lymph nodes are the inguinal nodes, the common iliac nodes, and the para-aortic nodes.

N0: No evidence of regional lymph node involvement.
N1: Evidence of involvement of a single homolateral regional lymph node.
N2: Evidence of involvement of contralateral or bilateral or multiple regional lymph nodes.
N3: Evidence of involvement of fixed regional lymph nodes (there is a fixed mass on the pelvic wall with a free space between this and the tumour).
N4: Evidence of involvement of juxtaregional lymph nodes.
Note: If lymphography indicates extension to the juxtaregional lymph nodes, a scalene node biopsy is recommended.
NX: The minimum requirements for assessment of the regional and/or juxtaregional lymph nodes cannot be met.

M: Distant metastases.

M0: No evidence of distant metastases.
M1: Evidence of distant metastases.
MX: The minimum requirements for assessment of the presence of distant metastases cannot be met.

pTNM Postsurgical Histopathological Classification

pT: Primary tumour.

pTis: Pre-invasive carcinoma (carcinoma in situ).
pT0: No evidence of tumour found on histological examination of specimen.
pT1: Focal (single or multiple) carcinoma.
pT2: Diffuse carcinoma with or without extension to the capsule.
pT3: Carcinoma with invasion beyond the capsule and/or invasion of the seminal vesicles.
pT4: Tumour with invasion of adjacent organs.
pTX: The extent of tumour cannot be assessed.

G: Histopathological grading.

G1: High degree of differentiation.
G2: Medium degree of differentiation.
G3 Low degree of differentiation or undifferentiated.
GX: Grade cannot be assessed.

pN: Regional and juxtaregional lymph nodes.

The pN categories correspond to the N categories.

pM: Distant metastases.

The pM categories correspond to the M categories.

Stage Grouping. No stage grouping is recommended at present.

Table 3. Relationship between tumour stage, grade and size, presence of lymph node metastases, and subsequent development of metastases. Barzell et al. (1977)

	Positive lymph nodes (%)	Subsequent metastases (%)
Stage		
Confined within prostate (B)	15/59 (25)	8/59 (13)
Extension beyond prostate (C)	26/41 (63)	16/41 (40)
Grade		
Well differentiated	3/19 (16)	2/29 (10)
Moderately well-differentiated	18/46 (39)	8/56 (17)
Poorly differentiated	9/15 (60)	7/15 (47)
Size (cc)		
< 2.5	1/18 (5)	1/18 (5)
2.5–7.9	17/50 (34)	10/50 (20)
8–18	23/32 (72)	13/32 (41)
Total	41/100	24/100

Table 4. Incidence and site of nodal metastases in 15 patients. Golimbu et al. (1979)

External iliac	9 (60%)
Obturator	8 (53%)
Presacral	8 (53%)
Presciatic	7 (47%)
Common iliac	4 (27%)
Hypogastric	2 (14%)
External iliac/obturator	13 (86%)
Presacral/presciatic	12 (80%)

4 Detection of Lymph Node Metastases

Careful study of pelvic lymph nodes removed from patients with apparently localised prostatic carcinoma has revealed that up to 50% have contained metastases, and that subsequent development of distant spread was more likely, and the prognosis was worse, in patients with such metastases. Analysis of 100 consecutive cases by Barzell et al. (1977) showed that lymph node metastases were present in 41 patients, and that local extension, large size, and poor histological differentiation were all associated with an increased likelihood of lymph node involvement and of subsequent appearance of metastases (Table 3). Recognition that more accurate staging was of significant prognostic value has led to a more intensive search for metastases in many centres.

For example, Paulson et al. (1979) found that the addition of radio-isotopic bone scanning, lymphography, and pelvic lymph node dissection to the routine physical examination, skeletal survey and serum acid phosphatase produced 'up-staging' in between 26% and 57% of 454 patients. The technique of extended pelvic lymphadenectomy has been well described and illustrated by Golimbu and Morales

Table 5. Comparison of results of lymphography and lymphadenectomy

Reference	Lymphogram	Lymphadenectomy	
		Positive	Negative
O'Donoghue et al. (1976)	Positive	2	1
	Negative	4	13 (76%)
Loening et al. (1977)	Positive	12 (41%)	17
	Negative	4	7 (64%)
Paulson et al. (1979)	Positive	18 (90%)	2
	Negative	16	57 (78%)

(1980), and the distribution of involved pelvic nodes defined by Golimbu et al. (1979); see Table 4.

Whether lymphography could take the place of lymph node dissection is open to question. Comparative studies have shown that microscopic lymph node metastases should be expected in about 25% of patients with negative lymphograms (Table 5). The incidence of false-positive results has varied widely, and probably reflects the skill brought to the interpretation of the radiological changes (this volume, Chap. 7). Certainly, lymphography can provide unequivocal evidence of lymph node involvement which would not have been suspected on clinical examination (Fig. 4). The incidence of positive lymphograms increases with increasing stage of the disease (Table 6; Zingg et al. 1974), in the same way as the incidence of positive nodes on histological examination (see above).

The choice between lymphogram and lymphadenectomy to provide information on the pelvic nodes in patients with apparently localised disease is not particularly easy. Lymphadenectomy often produces some oedema, and deep venous thrombosis and pulmonary embolus have been observed after this procedure. Evidence derived from microscopic examination of tissue is bound to be more accurate than naked-eye

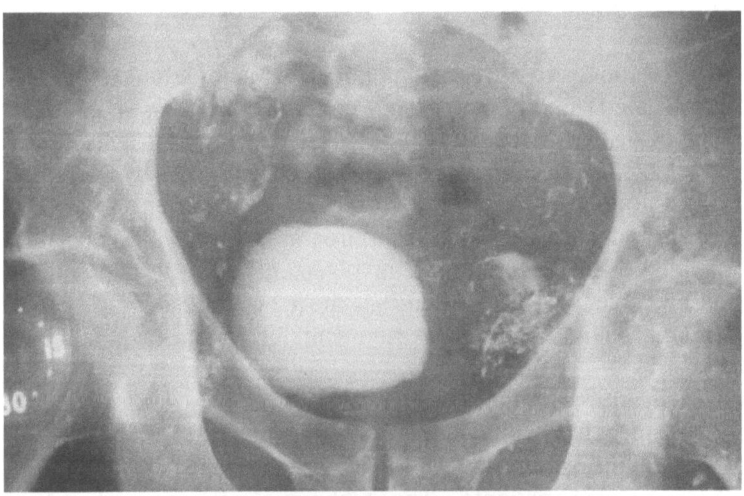

Fig. 4. Lymphogram showing massive involvement of pelvic nodes

Table 6. Incidence of lymph node metastases discovered by lymphography related to extent of primary tumour. Zingg et al. (1974)

Stage	Number of patients	Lymphogram	
		Negative	Positive
T0, T1	7	6	1
T2	19	12	7
T3, T4	34	11	23
Total	60	29	31

Table 7. C factor or level of certainty. UICC (1978)

C1	Evidence from clinical examination only
C2	Evidence obtained by special diagnostic means
C3	Evidence from surgical exploration only
C4	Evidence following definitive surgery
C5	Evidence from autopsy

Table 8. Incidence of lymph node metastases related to stage and grade of tumour[a] and acid phosphatase. Freiha et al. (1979)

Risk	Stage	Grade	Acid phos.	Positive nodes/ no. of patients
Low	A2, B1, B2	I, II, III	Normal	2/28 (7%)
Intermediate	A2	II	Elevated	21/58 (36%)
	B	I, II, III	Elevated	
	C	I, II	Normal	
	C	I, II	Elevated	
High	C	III	Elevated	13/14 (93%)

[a] American Joint Committee on Staging

examination of lymph nodes – either grossly or radiologically. This difference in accuracy can be expressed as the level of certainty, or C factor (Table 7). From a computation of other factors, such as stage, grade, and acid phosphatase, the probability of lymph node metastases can be estimated with a high degree of accuracy (Table 8) without the morbidity associated with surgical exploration. It seems likely that by combining lymphography with the known probability factors outlined above, the possibility of lymph node metastases may be judged with reasonable accuracy in planning management. The possible existence of microscopic deposits in pelvic lymph nodes should not be overlooked even when the lymphogram is normal.

Table 9. Survival after radical prostatectomy

Reference	No. of patients	Percentage surviving	
		10 years	15 years
Vickery and Kerr (1963)	65	58.5	–
	20	15.0	–
Mellinger et al. (1967)	85	38	–
	94	39	–
Berlin et al. (1968)	143	52	33
Jewett et al. (1972)	103	50	35
Culp and Meyer (1973)	115	72	–
	74	–	54
Veenema et al. (1977)	159	55	45

Table 10. Complications of radical prostatectomy. Veenema et al. (1977)

	Patients
Death	4 (2.5%)
Pulmonary emboli	6 (3.7%)
Stricture	29 (17%)
Incontinence	20 (12.5%)
Rectal injury	13 (7%)
Faecal fistula	3 (2.5%)
Osteitis pubis	1 (0.6%)
Total	159

5 Surgical Treatment

The surgeon must consider the possible role of radical prostatectomy in the management of early localised carcinoma. The reported survival rates are good (Table 9), although the list of complications is formidable (Table 10). It should be remembered that with small well-differentiated tumours, the 10-year survival rate is similar to that of men of the same age distribution in the general population (Bauer et al. 1960). Blackard et al. (1971) have shown no significant differences in focal carcinoma between patients who received no therapy (45 patients), hormonal therapy (22 patients), or radical prostatectomy (24 patients). Barnes and Ninan (1972) reported 10- and 15-year survival rates of 60% and 36%, respectively, with endocrine therapy and with TUR if necessary in patients with early localised disease. Excellent results have been reported with radiotherapy, especially with iodine-125 implantation and pelvic lymphadenectomy (Witmore et al. 1979; this volume, Chap. 10).
Further clinical trials are clearly needed to establish the optimum treatment for patients with prostatic carcinoma, stratified according to the extent of the disease. Such trials are now being conducted by the Medical Research Council for early (T0, T1) and more advanced (T2, T3, and T4) tumours with no evidence of distant metastases (M0) (this volume, Chap. 12).

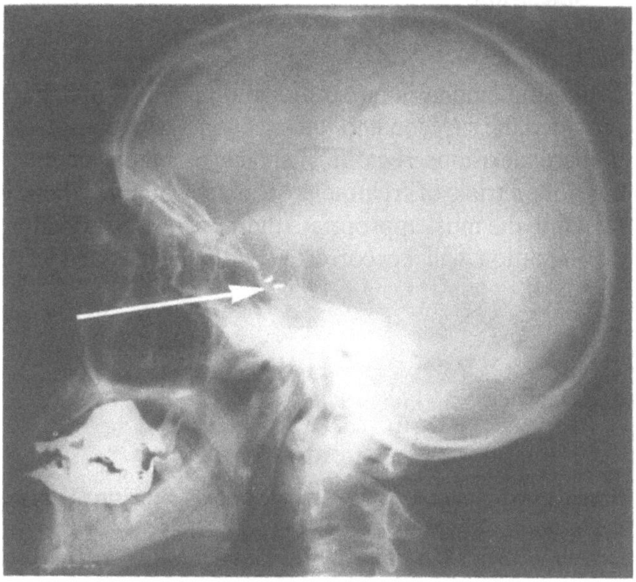

Fig. 5. Pituitary ablation by implantation of radioactive yttrium needles

6 Endocrine Ablation

Castration lowers the plasma testosterone as effectively as stilboestrol 1 mg t.d.s. (Shearer et al. 1973), and subcapsular orchidectomy is as effective as total orchidectomy (Clark and Houghton 1977). Early studies suggested that orchidectomy gave marginally better results than oestrogens (Nesbit and Baum 1950; Emmett et al. 1960), but subsequent studies by the Veterans Administration failed to show significant differences although there were far fewer cardiovascular deaths after orchidectomy (Veterans Administration Co-operative Urological Research Group 1967). Recognition of the side effects associated with oestrogens, including gynaecomastia, cardiovascular problems, and depression, has produced a swing towards orchidectomy once again, and this method of primary endocrine therapy has been chosen for the MRC trial in advanced local disease.

Although most patients with disseminated disease derive considerable benefit from endocrine therapy, many eventually relapse and their management then presents many problems. Mahoney and Harrison (1972) and others (reviewed by Hendry 1974) have shown that up to 80% of patients may derive some subjective benefit from bilateral adrenalectomy, although objective evidence of remission is much less common. This is a major operation to inflict upon a patient already ill with disseminated cancer, and there is good evidence that almost as good results can be obtained by medical suppression of the adrenals with cortisone 37.5–50 mg daily (Miller and Hinman 1954; Birke et al. 1955) or with aminoglutethimide (Robinson et al. 1974). Pituitary ablation by surgical hypophysectomy or cryosurgery (Murphy et al. 1971) may produce improvement in rather more than half the patients treated, but this objective is more easily achieved by implantation with radioactive yttrium-90 needles (Fig. 5). Fergusson and Hendry (1971) described complete and lasting relief of pain in 39, and partial relief in 32, of 100 patients treated by this method.

7 Conclusions

Increasing emphasis on accuracy in diagnosis and staging of prostatic carcinoma has provided the surgeon and the oncologist with considerably more information on which to base decisions regarding choice of management. Until the results of carefully controlled trials of treatment become available, there is little to guide the surgeon in selecting the most appropriate therapy for the individual patient. It is to be hoped that this situation will be corrected with the passage of time.

8 References

Barnes RW, Ninan CA (1972) Carcinoma of the prostate: biopsy and conservative therapy. J Urol 108: 897–900

Barzell W, Bean MA, Hilaris BS, Whitmore WF (1977) Prostatic adenocarcinoma: relationship of grade and local extent to the pattern of metastases. J Urol 118: 278–282

Bauer WC, McGarvan MH, Carlin MR (1960) Unsuspected carcinoma of the prostate in suprapubic prostatectomy specimens. Cancer 13: 370–378

Berlin BB, Cornwell PM, Connelly RR, Eisenberg H (1968) Radical perineal prostatectomy for carcinoma of the prostate: survival in 143 cases treated from 1935–1958. J Urol 99: 97–101

Birke G, Franksson C, Plantin LO (1955) Steroid response to hormone therapy in prostatic cancer. Acta Chir Scand 109: 129–149

Blackard CE, Mellinger GT, Gleason DF (1971) Treatment of stage 1 carcinoma of the prostate: a preliminary report. J Urol 106: 729–733

Chilton CP, Morgan RJ, England HR, Paris AMI, Blandy JP (1978) A critical evaluation of the results of transurethral resection of the prostate. Br J Urol 50: 542–546

Clark P, Houghton L (1977) Subcapsular orchidectomy for carcinoma of the prostate. Br J Urol 49: 419–425

Culp OS, Meyer JJ (1973) Radical prostatectomy in the treatment of prostatic cancer. Cancer 32: 1113–1118

Daves JA, Tomskey GC, Cohen AE (1961) Transrectal needle biopsy of the prostate. J Urol 85: 180–182

Denton SE, Valk WL, Jacobson JM, Kettunen RC (1967) Comparison of the perineal needle biopsy and the transurethral prostatectomy in the diagnosis of prostatic carcinoma: an analysis of 300 cases. J Urol 97: 127–129

Emmett JL, Greene LF, Papantoniou A (1960) Endocrine therapy in carcinoma of the prostate gland: 10 year survival studies. J Urol 83: 471–484

Fergusson JD, Hendry WF (1971) Pituitary irradiation in advanced carcinoma of the prostate: analysis of 100 cases. Br J Urol 43: 514–519

Franzén S, Giertz G, Zajicek J (1960) Cytological diagnosis of prostatic tumours by transrectal aspiration biopsy: a preliminary report. Br J Urol 32: 193–196

Freiha FS, Pistenma DA, Bagshaw MA (1979) Pelvic lymphadenectomy for staging prostatic carcinoma: is it always necessary? J Urol 122: 176–177

Golimbu M, Morales P (1979) Stage A_2 prostatic carcinoma – should the staging system be reclassified? Urology 13: 592–596

Golimbu M, Morales P (1980) Extended pelvic lymphadenectomy. Urology 15: 298–301

Golimbu M, Morales P, Al-Askari S, Brown J (1979) Extended pelvic lymphadenectomy for prostatic cancer. J Urol 121: 617–620

Hendry WF (1974) Adrenalectomy and hypophysectomy in disseminated prostatic cancer. In: Castro JE (ed) The treatment of prostatic hypertrophy and neoplasia. Medical and Technical Publishing, Lancaster, pp 171–196
Hendry WF, Williams JP (1971) Transrectal prostatic biopsy. Br Med J 4: 595–597
Jewett HJ, Eggleston JC, Yawn DH (1972) Radical prostatectomy in the management of carcinoma of the prostate: probable causes of some therapeutic failures. J Urol 107: 1034–1040
Lennox EL, Stiller CA, Morris Jones PH, Kinnier Wilson LM (1979) Nephroblastoma: treatment during 1970-3 and the effect on survival of inclusion in the first MRC trial. Br Med J 2: 567–569
Loening SA, Schmidt JD, Brown RC, Hawtrey CE, Fallon B, Culp DA (1977) A comparison between lymphangiography and pelvic node dissection in the staging of prostatic cancer. J Urol 117: 752–756
Mahoney EM, Harrison JH (1972) Bilateral adrenalectomy for palliative treatment of prostatic cancer. J Urol 108: 936–938
Mellinger GT, Gleason DF,Bailar J III (1967) The histology and prognosis of prostatic cancer. J Urol 97: 331–337
Miller GM, Himan F (1954) Cortisone treatment in advanced carcinoma of the prostate. J Urol 72: 485–496
Murphy GP, Reynoso G, Schoonees R, Gailani S, Bourke R, Kenny GM, Mirand EA, Schalch DS (1971) Hypophysectomy and adrenalectomy for disseminated prostatic carcinoma. J Urol 105: 817–825
Nesbit RM, Baum WC (1950) Endocrine control of prostatic carcinoma: clinical and statistical survey of 1818 cases. JAMA 143: 1317–1320
O'Donoghue EPN, Pugh RCB (1977) Early diagnosis of prostatic carcinoma: the role of transurethral resection. Br J Urol 49: 705–710
O'Donoghue EPN, Shridhar P, Sherwood T, Williams JP, Chisholm GD (1976) Lymphography and pelvic lymphadenectomy in carcinoma of the prostate. Br J Urol 48: 689–696
Paulson DF, Uro-Oncology Research Group (1979) The impact of current staging procedures in assessing disease extent of prostatic adenocarcinoma. J Urol 121: 300–302
Peeling WB, Griffiths GJ, Evans RT, Roberts EE (1979) Diagnosis and staging of prostatic cancer by transrectal ultrasonography. A preliminary study. Br J Urol 51: 565–569
Purser BN, Robinson BC, Mostofi FK (1967) Comparison of needle biopsy and transurethral resection biopsy in the diagnosis of carcinoma of the prostate. J Urol 98: 224–228
Robinson MRG, Shearer RJ, Fergusson JD (1974) Adrenal suppression in the treatment of carcinoma of prostate. Br J Urol 46: 555–559
Shearer RJ, Hendry WF, Sommerville IF, Fergusson JD (1973) Plasma testosterone: an accurate monitor of hormone treatment in prostatic cancer. Br J Urol 45: 668–677
UICC (1978) TNM Classification of Malignant Tumours, 3rd edn. UICC, Geneva
Veenema RJ, Gursel EO, Lattimer JK (1977) Radical retropubic prostatectomy for cancer: a 20-year experience. J Urol 117: 330–331
Veterans Administration Co-operative Urological Research Group (1967) Treatment and survival of patients with cancer of the prostate. Surg. Gynecol Obstet 124: 1011–1017
Vickery AL, Kerr WS (1963) Cancer of the prostate treated by radical prostatectomy: a clinicopathological survey of 187 cases followed for 5 years and 148 cases followed for 10 years. Cancer 16: 1598–1608
Whitmore WF, Batata M, Hilaris B (1979) Prostatic irradiation: Iodine-125 implantation. In: Johnson DE, Samuels ML (eds) Cancer of the genitourinary tract. Raven Press, New York, pp 195–205
Zingg EJ, Fuchs WA, Heritier P, Gothlin J (1974) Lymphography in carcinoma of the prostate. Br J Urol 46: 549–554

Radiotherapy

H. J. G. Bloom

Department of Radiotherapy and Oncology, Royal Marsden Hospital,
Institute of Cancer Research, GB – London SW3

1 Introduction

The aim of this chapter is to review the role of radical radiotherapy in the primary treatment of adenocarcinoma of the prostate. There has been little change in the application of various irradiation techniques for palliative treatment of this disease, and these have been considered elsewhere (Bloom and Hendry 1973).
Early experience with megavoltage irradiation, which was introduced in the 1950s, demonstrated that the reputation of radio-resistance in prostatic cancer was fallacious. Subsequent developments indicated that local control of the primary tumour could be obtained in a high proportion of patients without prohibitive acute local reactions or unacceptable late morbidity.
In addition to megavoltage beam treatment, which has been used with increasing frequency for cancer of the prostate over the past 10–15 years, there has also been a revival of interest in interstitial techniques in which gold-198 is used in colloidal form or as seeds and, more recently, in the use of iridium-192 wire and iodine-125 capsules.

2 Interstitital Irradiation

Just after World War II and prior to the megavoltage era, Flocks et al. (1952) began to use colloidal radiogold for interstitial irradiation in patients with prostatic cancer. These workers have treated over 1,000 patients, mainly with limited extraprostatic invasion (Flocks 1969). Other radiocolloids, such as chromic phosphate (P32) and yttrium chloride (Y90), have also been used for this purpose. All these isotopes are injected directly into the tumour or into the tumour bed after a preliminary debulking procedure. Flocks reported 5- and 10-year survival rates of 54% and 38%, respectively, with few complications (Flocks 1969; Rubin 1969).
General experience with radio-isotope colloids has been unsatisfactory, however, and Howe et al. (1963) report a high incidence of postoperative sequelae (18 of 22 cases). Because of the technical difficulty in achieving a satisfactory dose distribution with liquid isotopes, the possible risk of tumour cell dissemination in the blood stream resulting from increasing the intraprostatic pressure, and the frequent escape of the injected gold from the tumour, we chose to use solid radiogold sources inserted

Recent Results in Cancer Research, Vol. 78
© Springer-Verlag Berlin · Heidelberg 1981

transvesically into the tumour with the Royal Marsden Hospital repeating gun. Sixteen patients were treated by this technique just prior to the general availability in our centre of megavoltage equipment. There was one postoperative death. Of the remaining 15 patients, good local control of the disease was achieved in 11 (73%), in three patients for 5 or more years, in two patients for 2–3 years and in six patients until death. The 5-year survival rate was 38% (Bloom and Hendry 1973). This method of interstitial irradiation was quick and simple and presented less of a radiation hazard to operator and to staff than the injection of liquid isotopes. In addition, a more uniform irradiation was achieved in the tumour from the gamma rays emitted by the solid gold-198 sources than with the predominantly beta-ray component from colloidal material of the isotope.

In spite of the general availability of megavoltage equipment at present for the treatment of deep-seated tumours, the principle of intensive local interstitial irradiation for primary prostatic tumours of limited size, with sparing of surrounding normal tissues, remains an attractive proposition. Court and Chassagne (1977) have used an after-loading technique with iridium-192 wires in carefully selected patients with T1 and T2 tumours and without node involvement. Carlton et al. (1975) and also Chan and Gutierrez (1976) combined local irradiation by means of gold-198 grains with external beam therapy and reported promising early results. Whitmore and his group (Whitmore et al. 1972, 1979; Hilaris et al. 1977) have also used an after-loading technique to deliver low-energy irradiation from the slow-decaying isotope iodine-125 in selected cases, including many with clinical extraprostatic spread.

The chief advantage of iodine-125 is the low-energy irradiation, which results in negligible exposure of staff. It is not yet known whether the protracted irradiation resulting from the permanent implants of this low-energy-emitting isotope has any biological advantage over the more intense, shorter-term high-energy irradiation from gold-198 sources. Gold-198, as a permanent implant, with a short half-life of 2.7 days, delivers a dose of between 6,500 and 7,000 rads, mostly within the first few days. In the case of iodine-125, with a half-life of 60 days, the total dose of 16,000 rads is delivered over 1 year, 8,000 rads being reached in the first 2 months. It is postulated that this type of protracted irradiation may be an advantage for the control of slow-growing tumours. For long half-life isotopes with high-energy radiations, such as tantalum-182, the sources must be removed, generally after a dose of between 6,000 and 6,500 rads in 6–7 days.

Hilaris et al. (1977) reported encouraging early experience in 208 patients treated with iodine-125 seeds combined with lymphadenectomy. The nodes were histologically positive in 29% of 128 stage B cases, and 59% of 80 stage C cases. The crude 5-year survival rate for 26 patients followed up for 5 years was 70%. It was 100% for six stage B cases and 63% for 20 stage C cases. Of 13 patients with negative nodes, 94% were still alive, compared with 48% of those with positive nodes. Although the overall 5-year survival rate for interstitial irradiation in node-positive cases at first appears to be encouraging (20/37; 54%), the true picture should be judged by 'survival without evidence of disease', and at 5 years this was only 19% (7/37) in the Memorial Hospital series (Whitmore et al. 1979).

Interstitital irradiation appears to offer a simpler alternative to radical prostatectomy for small, strictly limited, and more differentiated tumours. The surgical and irradiation morbidity is low and impotence is a rare sequel in previously potent men. Patients with large, less well-differentiated lesions are unsuitable for an implant, because of the difficulty of obtaining a uniform dose distribution and of including all suspected lines of direct and lymphatic tumour extension within the treated volume. For such cases external beam therapy appears to be a more logical approach to radical treatment.

The general limitations of interstitial therapy call for a careful selection of patients with localised disease for this type of treatment. Court and Chassagne (1977) recommend using implants of iridium-192 wire only for stage T1 and T2 cases without lymph node involvement, based on ilio-obturator lymphadenectomy and immediate frozen section examination. Other workers have been less selective in their choice of cases for interstitial irradiation and have included some patients with extraprostatic spread as well as cases with proven lymph node involvement (Whitmore et al. 1979).

Lymph node sampling or dissection in patients to be treated by interstitial irradiation has provided useful information regarding tumour extent and prognosis. Pelvic lymphadenectomy alone, however, cannot be expected to control substantial regional disease for long, and node-positive cases will undoubtedly need additional treatment which, at present, is probably best provided by supplementary large-volume external beam irradiation (Whitmore et al. 1979) (Tables 1 and 2). However, the benefit of this additional treatment has yet to be firmly established. Almost 70% of patients with positive nodes develop bone metastases within 5 years of treatment, compared with 31% of those with negative nodes (Hilaris et al. 1977).

Table 1. Carcinoma of the prostate treated by iodine-125 implant with or without supplementary external beam irradiation at the Memorial Hospital. Disease-free survival rates by clinical stage in node-positive patients. Five-year results are based on 37 patients. Whitmore et al. (1979)

Stage	Patients	Alive NED	
		2 years (%)	5 years (%)
T1	11	45	0
T2	20	65	33
T3	22	50	37
T4	36	33	14
Total	89	46	19

Table 2. Carcinoma of prostate treated by iodine-125 implant with or without supplementary external beam irradiation at the Memorial Hospital. Disease-free survival rates by treated volume in node-positive patients. Five-year results based on 37 patients. Whitmore et al. (1978)

External irradiation	Patients	Alive NED	
		2 years (%)	5 years (%)
Nil	65	47	21
Pelvis	14	43	0
Pelvis + para-aortic	10	40	25

3 Megavoltage Beam Therapy

Since the early observations reported from the United States by Bagshaw et al. (1965), George et al. (1965), and Del Regato (1967), and also from England by Budhraja and Anderson (1964), there has been increasing interest in the treatment of prostatic cancer by megavoltage external beam therapy.

Budhraja and Anderson (1964), in a non-randomised study, compared results in 53 histologically proven advanced cases of prostatic cancer treated by a combination of surgery, irradiation, and stilboestrol with those obtained in 28 cases treated by surgery and stilboestrol. The radiotherapy series included patients treated with the aid of a 2 MeV Van de Graaf generator. Twenty-six of 36 patients (72%) treated with megavoltage irradiation were alive at 3 years, compared with only 12 of 28 patients (43%) in the non-radiotherapy group. At 5 years, however, the results obtained in the two treatment groups were comparable. The absence of serious radiotherapy complications in this early study was particularly encouraging.

The major contribution to the subject of external beam therapy for prostatic cancer has undoubtedly been made by the Stanford University group. Their latest report contains over 500 patients (Bagshaw 1978), who have been divided into two groups. The first consists of 370 patients treated prior to 1971 by small-volume irradiation localised to the prostate and periprostatic tissue without prior surgical staging. The 5- and 10-year actuarial survival rates for 193 patients with disease clinically confined to the prostate (stage B) were 75% and 47%, respectively: of 177 patients with extraprostatic spread (stage C), 52% were alive at 5 years and 28% at 10 years (Table 3).

In the second group of the Stanford series there were 166 patients treated since 1971 by extended-field irradiation after more accurate selection, including lymph node sampling or dissection. So far, the overall survival and disease-free survival of patients with stage B and C tumours, many of whom had positive nodes, approximates closely to that for the patients in the previous group, in which the disease was clinically confined to the prostate (B) and who were treated by small-volume irradiation. This suggests that somc measure of regional tumour control has been achieved by the larger-volume treatment.

Some 5- and 10-year survival rates reported for patients with locally advanced carcinoma of the prostate (T3–T4; C) are shown in Table 4.

The degree of local tumour control following external beam therapy is an important consideration when the value of radiotherapy is assessed. McGowan (1977) reported

Table 3. Carcinoma of prostate treated by small-volume external beam irradiation. Total and disease-free survival rates (actuarial) by clinical stage at Stanford University. Bagshaw (1978)

Stage	Patients	Alive 5 years		Alive 10 years	
		Total (%)	NED (%)	Total (%)	NED (%)
B	193	75	67	47	47
C	177	52	44	28	33
Total	370	63	–	40	–

Table 4. Carcinoma of prostate treated by external beam irradiation. Reported survival rates at 5 and 10 years in stage C (T3–T4) cancer

Reference	Patients	Alive	
		5 years (%)	10 years (%)
Hill et al. (1974)	36	42	31
Cantril et al. (1974)	180	42	–
Pistenna et al. (1976)	200	41	31
Perez et al. (1977)	97	42	–
Harisiadis et al. (1978)	112	58	–

Table 5. Carcinoma of prostate treated by external beam irradiation (6,000 rads/6 weeks). Disease-free survival rate (actuarial) by clinical stage at Edmonton/Calgary Cancer Clinics. McGowan (1977)

Stage	Patients	5-Year survival (NED) (%)
A	21	84
B1	43	61
B2	30	43
C	13	37
Total	107	74

complete clinical resolution in 78 of 86 patients (91%) with B1 to C tumours following a dose of 6,000 rads in 6 weeks. The overall 5-year disease-free survival rate in this series was 74%, ranging from 84% for stage A to 37% for stage C cases (Table 5). Local failure occurred in only 12% of patients in the Stanford study (Pistenma et al. 1976) and in 9% of 23 five-year survivors reported by Hill et al. (1974). In a review of seven series in the literature, covering 797 collected cases, Cox and Stoffel (1977) found local recurrence in only 13%.

4 Prostatic Biopsy after Radiotherapy

Long-term, disease-free survival rates following external beam irradiation are being reported with increasing frequency. However, clouding the optimism over this type of treatment is the high incidence of positive prostatic biopsies found some months after completion of radiotherapy. Various authors have reported incidences of residual tumour ranging from 14% (George et al. 1965) to as high as 87% (Rhamy et al. 1972). The average among 57 biopsied cases collected from the literature was 46% (Bloom and Hendry 1973).

It now appears that a single positive biopsy may lack significance since, with the passage of time, it may become negative. Cox and Stoffel (1977) reported their

Table 6. Incidence of positive biopsies in 38 patients with stage C carcinoma of prostate at various intervals following radiotherapy (7,000 rads/ 6 weeks). Cox and Stoffel (1977)

Interval (months)	Patients	+ ve Biopsy (%)
6	29	16 (55)
12	31	12 (39)
18	26	8 (31)
30	37	7 (19)
42	16	3 (19)

Table 7. Local tumour recurrence following radiotherapy for carcinoma of prostate in 797 collected cases from 13 reports. Incidence of positive biopsies within 1 year and after 1 year following treatment. Cox and Stoffel (1977)

	Incidence (%)
Local recurrence	106/797 (13)
+ ve Biopsy ≤ 1 year	84/133 (63)
+ ve Biopsy > 1 year	80/175 (46)

experience with 38 stage C patients treated with 7,000 rads in 6–7 weeks in whom post-therapy serial biopsies were carried out for up to 42 months. Positive specimens were obtained in 55% of 29 patients at 6 months, 39% of 31 patients at 12 months and by 30 months only 19% of 37 patients still had tumour present (Table 6). Cox and Stoffel (1977) also reviewed the literature, and found that residual tumour was reported in 63% of 133 collected cases biopsied within 1 year of radiotherapy, compared with 46% of 175 patients in whom the biopsies were delayed for more than a year (Table 7).

It is important to appreciate that histopathological tumour regression can be very slow in cancer of the prostate, that sampling errors may occur in biopsy specimens, and that even late positive biopsies may not necessarily indicate the presence of viable cells capable of progressive division. Nevertheless, a persistently positive biopsy after a year following external beam irradiation tends to be associated with a poorer prognosis than negative biopsies (Cosgrove and Kaemf 1976; Perez et al. 1977).

Nachtsheim et al. (1978) studied serial needle biopsies from 50 patients treated by megavoltage irradiation (6,500 rads to prostate and 4,500 rads to pelvic nodes). Of 29 biopsies taken 18 or more months after treatment, 15 (52%) contained carcinoma. Of 17 taken after 36 months, 10 (59%) were still positive (Table 8). The authors concluded that patients with residual tumour 18 months after treatment are not expected to show resolution in the future and should be regarded as treatment failures.

No satisfactory correlation has yet been demonstrated between clinical progress and the interpretation of postirradiation biopsy findings. Further studies with prolonged follow-up are required.

Table 8. Incidence of posttreatment positive biopsies within 18 months, after 18 months, and after 36 months. If biopsy is positive at 18 months there appears to be no further resolution. Nachtsheim et al. (1978)

Interval (months)	Patients	Residual tumour (%)
< 18	21	6 (29)
≥ 18	29	15 (52)
≥ 36	17	10 (59)

If residual cancer cells at the primary site following external beam therapy for prostatic cancer are significant and an important cause of local failure and tumour spread, more intensive local irradiation, which can be achieved by interstitial techniques alone or in combination with external beam therapy, may play an important role in the management of the primary disease. However, a recent study (Guerriero et al. 1979) revealed that following a combination of gold-198 implantation (3,000–3,500 rads) and megavoltage irradiation (4,000–5,000 rads), posttreatment biopsies at 1 year were still positive in 38% of 21 patients with stage A tumours, in 35% of 43 stage B cases, in 38% of 45 stage C1 cases, and in 56% of 27 stage D1 cases. These findings following the combined treatment do not appear to differ significantly from those after megavoltage irradiation alone.

5 Lymph Node Involvement and Treatment Policy

In the past, attention has been focussed mainly on the progress of the primary tumour and on the development of blood-borne metastases in patients with prostatic cancer. In more recent years there has been increasing interest in lymphatic involvement with regard to frequency, pattern of spread, and possible means of control. The lymphatic system is frequently involved in prostatic cancer, and this raises the question as to whether this complication is purely incidental to concomitant blood spread and the inevitable harbinger of bony metastases. Whilst this is probably true for the majority of patients with para-aortic node deposits, it is not necessarily so for patients with disease limited to the pelvic nodes. In such cases lymphadenectomy and external beam irradiation may be of value.

5.1 Lymphographic Assessment

The results of bilateral pedal lymphography in 83 patients with prostatic cancer were reported from the Royal Marsden Hospital by Paxton et al. (1975). Sixty-five percent had positive lymphograms. Of 24 patients with T0–T2 disease, 37% were positive, compared with 76% of 59 patients with T3–T4 lesions. In 17 new patients with early lesions (T1 and T2) the lymphogram was positive in 41%. Involvement of the

Table 9. Incidence of histologically positive nodes in patients with prostatic carcinoma according to stage. Note the high incidence in patients with clinically unsuspected diffuse carcinoma (A2). Donohue et al. (1979)

Stage	Patients	Histological + ve nodes (%)
A1	6	0 (0)
A2	27	8 (30)
B1	67	15 (22)
B2	21	12 (57)
Total	121	35 (29)

para-aortic nodes was seen in 23% of the total series. It is important to note that this complication was present in two of 15 patients with T2 tumours. Although the lymphographic findings in this series were not confirmed by histological studies, a high degree of accuracy was claimed by Paxton et al. (1975) on the grounds of careful follow-up X-ray films from which an increase in metastatic growth or a response to irradiation could be assessed.

Pedal lymphography may present false-positive results, fail to show metastases unless they are more than 0.5 cm in diameter (Koehler 1976) and, of course, will not opacify the obturator, internal iliac and sacrococcygeal nodes. About 25% of patients with negative lymphograms have histologically positive nodes. The overall accuracy rate for lymphography, based on lymphadenectomy studies, is between 75% and 85% (Cerny et al. 1975; O'Donoghue et al. 1976; Spellman et al. 1977).

5.2 Histological Assessment

Histological evidence of node involvement may be found in a substantial number of early cases of prostatic cancer. For example, Donohue et al. (1979) reported 30% of patients with clinically unsuspected diffuse prostatic cancer (stage A2) as having positive nodes, based on pelvic lymphadenectomy specimens (Table 9). Nodal metastases have been reported in 20%–40% of patients with clinical T1 and T2 (B) tumours. In T3 (C) cases the incidence is generally between 50% and 70% (McCullough et al. 1974; Dahl et al. 1974; McLaughlin et al. 1976; Hilaris et al. 1977; Spellman et al. 1977; Pistenma et al. 1979). The obturator nodes are the most frequently involved, followed by the external and internal iliac groups. Bilateral metastases may be seen as often as unilateral ones (Hilaris et al. 1977). Golimbu et al. (1979) have drawn attention to a high incidence of metastases in the presacral and presciatic node groups.

In view of these observations, strictly local treatment, such as that provided by interstitial techniques, has serious limitations even in the presence of early tumour extension beyond the prostate. External beam therapy, by providing uniform en bloc irradiation of the primary tumour, periprostatic tissue, and regional nodes, appears to represent a more suitable treatment than interstitial irradiation for the majority of patients with prostatic cancer without distant metastases.

6 External Beam Therapy

6.1 Tumour Dose

It is widely appreciated that high-dose irradiation is necessary to control prostatic cancer, and most authors recommend tumour doses in the range of 6,500–7,500 rads, fractionated daily over 6–8 weeks. The risks of such treatment depend chiefly on the volume of tissue irradiated, the number of fractions, and the overall time in which treatment is given. For example, if the whole true pelvis is to be irradiated, the dose should not exceed 5,000 rads: any additional treatment should be given as a boost to a strictly limited volume to bring the maximum primary tumour dose to 6,500–7,000 rads in an overall time of not less than 7 weeks. It is essential to protract such large-volume treatment over this period if serious early or late injuries are to be avoided.

Some authors have recommended maximum tumour doses as high as 7,000–7,500 rads, which undoubtedly carry an increased risk of serious damage to normal tissues. When Werf-Messing et al. (1976) reduced the tumour dose in their series from 7,000 rads in 7 weeks to 6,500–7,000 rads in 6.5–7 weeks, with or without a rest period after 4,000 rads, the complication rate was reduced from 23% (7/30) to 10% (3/30). Furthermore, it does not seem necessary to give more than 7,000 rads to the primary tumour, since high rates of clinical local tumour control (of the order of 90%) have been achieved with 6,000–7,000 rads. Harisiadis et al. (1978) reported local recurrence in only nine of 146 patients (6%) after such doses, and McGowan (1977) achieved local control with 6,000 rads in 91% of 86 cases. Harisiadis et al. (1978) report a 5-year survival rate of 87% following doses of 6,500–7,000 rads, compared with 57% for doses of 5,000–6,500 rads (mostly 6,000–6,500 rads). Hussey (1979) found local control and survival rates following 6,500 rads in 6.5 weeks to be comparable to those following 7,000 rads in 7–7.5 weeks for both stage B and stage C1 cases. However, for patients with C2 tumours (i.e., massive growth with fixation to one or both pelvic walls or invasion of adjacent organs) the higher dose of 7,000 rads gave better results, but at the expense of significantly more complications (Table 10). In general, it seems that we should aim to deliver a maximum tumour dose of between 6,500 and 7,000 rads in 7–8 weeks.

Table 10. Local tumour control, survival, and incidence of treatment complications by irradiation dose in patients with stage C (C1 and C2) carcinoma of prostate at M. D. Anderson Hospital. Minimum follow-up 4 years. Hussey (1979)

Stage	Local control		Survival		Complications	
	6,500 (%)	7,000 (%)	6,500 (%)	7,000 (%)	6,500 (%)	7,000 (%)
C1	94	92	65	64	6	11
C2	62	79	31	56	0	12

6.2 *Treatment Volume*

Bagshaw et al. (1965) obtained their earlier encouraging results with small-volume, high-dose irradiation restricted to the prostate and periprostatic tissue. No attempt was made specifically to treat the regional lymph nodes. Recent data regarding lymphatic spread of prostatic cancer has raised the question of whether treatment of pelvic nodes is likely to improve results. At one time it was felt that node involvement in prostatic cancer was simply a forerunner of blood-borne metastases. It now appears that quite extensive pelvic node deposits may exist, at least for a time, without skeletal or visceral metastases. Long-term control and perhaps even cure may be possible in some patients with limited pelvic node involvement following extended-field radiotherapy. In several reports an increase in irradiated volume has *not* been associated with an increase in 5-year survival rate (Hill et al. 1974; Lipsett et al. 1976; Harisiadis et al. 1978). It could be argued that if early regional node metastases can be controlled, this can be achieved by limited-volume treatment, whereas if the node involvement is at all extensive, control even by extended-field irradiation is unlikely to be successful. Pistenma et al. (1979) have recently reported their preliminary observations in 86 patients treated at Stanford University in a current trial to evaluate extended-field irradiation which included the next echelon of nodes beyond those obviously involved. Thus, if the tumour is confined to the primary site, treatment is given to the prostate and the periprostatic region, with randomized patients receiving additional prophylactic pelvic irradiation. If the pelvic nodes are involved, then treatment is given to the whole pelvis in every case and patients are randomized to receive prophylactic para-aortic node irradiation. If pelvic and para-aortic nodes are involved all cases receive treatment to both regions (Table 11). Of the node-negative patients, 76% (41/54) were alive between 15 months and 7 years after treatment without evidence of disease, compared with 28% (9/32) of those with positive nodes. Patients with negative nodes did not seem to benefit from extended-field irradiation which included all the pelvic nodes. Seven of 18 patients (39%) with positive pelvic nodes were alive and disease-free following such treatment. It is too early to say whether irradiation of the para-aortic nodes will give additional benefit. When the para-aortic nodes are involved the prognosis is generally very poor indeed, only two of 14 such patients (14%) being alive without evidence of disease: nine of the 14 patients (64%) developed bone metastases. Thus, 28% of all 32 patients with positive nodes in the Stanford series were

Table 11. Extended volume irradiation for carcinoma of prostate. Disease-free survival (15 months to 7 years) by node involvement and treatment volume at Stanford University. Pistenma et al. (1979)

Nodes	Treatment	Patients	Alive NED (%)
Negative pelvic	Prostate	26	21 (81)
	Pelvis	28	20 (71)
Positive pelvic	Pelvis	11	4 (36)
	Pelvis and para-aortic nodes	7	3 (43)
Positive pelvic and para-aortic	Pelvis and para-aortic nodes	14	2 (14)

alive with no clinical-radiological evidence of disease, 15 months to 7 years after extended-field irradiation: an additional three patients with positive prostatic biopsies were alive, making the overall survival rate for node-positive cases 37% (12/32). Charyulu et al. (1979) have recently also reported encouraging results following pelvic and para-aortic irradiation: eight of 17 patients (47%) with verified positive nodes were alive and well with a median disease-free survival of 3.5 years.

Although a high proportion of patients with extensive node involvement will develop skeletal metastases and therefore one cannot be too hopeful about the value of node irradiation in such cases, it would seem worthwhile continuing the studies of extended-volume treatment, especially in those cases in which metastases appear to be limited to pelvic nodes.

In spite of these considerations concerning nodal irradiation, good results for limited-volume irradiation in patients with prostatic cancer have been reported by Ray et al. (1973) and by Hussey (1979). Using tumour doses generally in the range of 6,000–7,000 rads in 6–7.5 weeks, with the final 1,000–2,000 rads given through reduced fields, Hussey (1979) obtained 5- and 10-year survival rates of 64% and 42%, respectively, for stage C cases. Local control was achieved in 84% and major complications occurred in 8%. Although the type of treatment reported by Hussey (1979) is regarded as limited-field irradiation and certainly excluded the higher node groups (common iliac), it often did include the periprostatic, obturator, and at least some of the internal iliac nodes. This is perhaps why 'regional without central' failure in the pelvic cavity was reported in only 3% (5/170) of Hussey's patients, and 'regional with or without central failure' in only 8% (13/170).

Although bilateral pedal lymphography is associated with 75%–80% accuracy, this investigation is limited to assessment of the state of the external iliac, common iliac, and para-aortic nodes. It does not demonstrate the immediate echelon of regional nodes in the obturator, internal iliac, and presacral groups. It is also important to remember that 20% of lymphograms give false-negative results. Hence, in patients with negative lymphograms and in those without histological information concerning node status, the volume of tissue to be treated will depend on the likelihood of node involvement, based on the size, extent, and histological grade of the primary tumour. It is essential to weigh possible advantages of large-volume irradiation, aimed at controlling lymph node metastases, against the increased morbidity and possible mortality of such treatment, and to select high-risk patients in whom additional therapeutic hazards would be justified. However, with increased fractionation and split-course techniques it is possible to achieve satisfactory large-volume treatment with a low morbidity (Pistenma et al. 1979).

For the present, extended-volume irradiation and lymphadenectomy must be regarded as experimental therapeutic procedures, the surgical approach also providing useful diagnostic information. Details of the node groups involved, the number and size of positive nodes, and the degree of histological involvement should, whenever possible, be carefully assessed, documented, and correlated with treatment policy and results.

6.3 Complications

Acute urinary and rectal symptoms during and immediately after external beam therapy are usually mild to moderate and generally subside within 3–4 weeks of completing treatment. Such local symptoms are to be expected in about one-third to one-half of patients (Odell et al. 1971; Pistenma et al. 1976; McGowan 1977) and do not constitute serious complications. Acute symptoms are severe in about 5% of patients and in about 12% they become chronic, lasting more than 3 months but generally resolving within a year. Serious late sequelae are infrequent and include urethral strictures, rectal ulceration and faecal or urinary stress incontinence (Table 12). These complications were seen in 5% of 430 patients in the Stanford series (Ray and Bagshaw 1975). Major non-fatal complications were also reported in 5% of 112 patients by Perez et al. (1977), and included three cases of proctitis and one each of small-bowel stricture, pubic bone necrosis, and perirectal abscess.

Postirradiation small-bowel injury is more likely to occur in patients with a history of previous abdominal surgery, and for this reason lymphadenectomy prior to external beam therapy should be performed extraperitoneally. In patients with previous abdominal operations, barium studies may help to identify those at special risk with adherent loops of small bowel in relation to the volume to be irradiated. Fixed bowel loops sometimes occur without a history of previous surgery (Green et al. 1978).

The incidence and severity of radiation sequelae depend upon dose fractionation, total dose, and volume irradiated. Hill et al. (1974), using large treatment fields and doses in the range of 6,500–7,500 rads, reported significant sequelae in 30% of 46 patients, even though the overall treatment time was extended over 7–11 weeks. When the large-volume dose was reduced to 4,000 rads and followed by a boost of 2,000–2,500 rads confined to the prostatic region (maximum tumour dose, 6,000–6,500 rads), complications were virtually eliminated.

In an effort to reduce disturbance and the risk of late sequelae following extended-field treatment which includes the para-aortic nodes, the Stanford group rearranged their irradiation schedule as follows. First, 2,600 rads were given to a large volume in 2.5 weeks. This was followed by a small volume boost to the prostate of 2,000 rads in 2 weeks, and finally large-volume treatment was resumed to deliver a further 2,400 rads in 2.5 weeks. Thus, 5,000 rads were given to the pelvis and para-aortic region and 7,000 rads to the prostate in an overall time of 7 weeks. Finally, the surgical approach to the regional nodes was changed from a transperitoneal to a retroperitoneal procedure. These modifications reduced the incidence of serious intestinal symptoms from 67% to 3% and the need for surgical intervention from 38% to 0% (Pistenma et al. 1979) (Table 13).

At one time it was thought that an advantage of external beam irradiation over radical prostatectomy or endocrine therapy would be preservation of sexual potency. However, Ray and Bagshaw (1975) reported reduced potency in 41% of 110 patients

Table 12. Incidence of complications following external beam irradiation

Reference	Patients	Complications (%)
Mollenkamp et al. (1975)	88	7 (8)
Perez et al. (1977)	112	6 (5)
Ray and Bagshaw (1975)	430	22 (5)
Neglia et al. (1977)	154	12 (8)
Werf-Messing et al. (1976)	60	10 (17)

Table 13. Incidence of small-bowel complications following extended-field radiotherapy for carcinoma of prostate at Stanford University (Pistenma et al. 1979). Note reduction in both serious symptoms and necessity for surgery with changes in irradiation schedule and surgical technique

Period	Patients	Serious symptoms (%)	Surgery required (%)
1971–1973[a]	21	14 (67)	8 (38)
1973–1975[b]	12	2 (17)	1 (8)
1975–1977[c]	30	1 (3)	0 (0)

[a] Transperitoneal node biopsy followed by 5,500 rads/5.5 weeks plus local prostate boost of 1,500 rads/1.5 weeks
[b] Transperitoneal node biopsy followed by 2,600 rads/2.5 weeks plus local prostate boost of 2,000 rads/1.2 weeks plus 2,400 rads/2.5 weeks making a maximum tumour dose of 7,000 rads/7 weeks
[c] Retroperitoneal node biopsy followed by irradiation schedule as described in previous footnote

in whom potency was present prior to radiotherapy and who did not receive endocrine manipulation. Rhamy et al. (1972) found impotence following external beam therapy in seven of 15 patients (47%) and Loh et al. (1971) reported this complication in no less than 16 of 19 patients (84%).

The causes of impaired sexual function are complex and often difficult to assess. After several weeks of external beam therapy directed to the genital region in a patient attending a cancer department daily, is it surprising that sexual potency may decrease further in men who are elderly, ill, worried, and already showing signs of such decline? A more detailed study is required to clarify the situation.

Following interstitial irradiation, with or without pelvic lymphadenectomy, sexual potency seems to be maintained in the vast majority of previously potent men (Herr 1979). This is in contrast to the 100% impotence rate following radical prostatectomy and perhaps up to 40% following external beam irradiation.

7 Factors Influencing Radiation Response and Prognosis

7.1 Histological Grade

Prognosis following radical megavoltage irradiation in patients with prostatic cancer can be correlated with the degree of tumour differentiation (Perez et al. 1977; de Muelenaere and Sandison 1976; Harisiadis et al. 1978). In the series studied by Perez et al. (1977), 65% of stage C patients with well-differentiated tumours were alive and disease-free at 5 years, compared with 50% of patients with moderately differentiated tumours and only 12% of those with poorly differentiated lesions within the same clinical stage (Table 14).

Table 14. Influence of histological tumour grade on local recurrence, distant metastases, and disease-free survival in patients with stage C carcinoma of prostate treated by external beam irradiation (22 MV) at Mallinckordt Institute. Perez et al. (1977)

Grade	Patients	Distant metastases only (%)	Local recurrence (%)	5-Year survival (NED) (%)
Well differentiated	33	9	12	65
Moderately differentiated	39	15	15	50
Poorly differentiated	25	48	32	12
Total	97	22	19	42

Tumours of lower-grade malignancy appear to show a greater response to irradiation than do high-grade lesions. Thus, Loh et al. (1971) found that 19 of 20 patients (95%) with intermediate-grade tumours became tumour-free after irradiation, in contrast to only four of 14 patients (29%) with high-grade lesions.

7.2 Clinical Stage of Primary Tumour

Not surprisingly, the more advanced lesions are less likely to be eradicated by irradiation. Loh et al. (1971) found that all of seven patients with tumours limited to the prostate became tumour-free, in contrast to only 16 of 28 patients (57%) in whom periprostatic invasion was present. Higher doses (7,000 rads) are required to achieve local control of the more advanced and bulky C2 lesions, compared with the 6,500-rad dose that appears to be adequate for the majority of B1 and C1 tumours (Hussey 1979).

7.3 Intravenous Pyelogram

The presence of obstructive changes in the pyelogram influences prognosis adversely. Harisiadis et al. (1978) report a 5-year survival rate of 24% for patients with this complication, compared with 71% for those in whom the pyelogram was normal.

7.4 Tumour Latency and Delay in Treatment

It is recognised that latent or incidentally found prostatic tumours do not necessarily progress to clinical cancer during the remaining lifetime of the host. In recent years, a view has been expressed that because of latency in prostatic cancer, treatment for some patients with early tumours may be deferred until there are clear signs of progression. In a recent controlled study organised by the Medical Research Council (unpublished work), one of the treatment arms for patients with T0 to T2 tumours was 'deferred therapy'. This concept must be carefully defined and assessed, since there is some evidence that a significant delay for patients with prostatic cancer may influence results of radical treatment adversely (Cantril et al. 1974; Perez et al. 1977; Harisiadis et al. 1978) (Table 15). Harisiadis et al. (1978) reported a 5-year survival rate of 70% among 120 patients starting radiotherapy within 6 months of diagnosis, in contrast to

Table 15. Effect of treatment delay on radiotherapy results. Five-year survival rates reported by various authors

Reference	Patients	Delay (months)			
		0–3 (%)	0–6 (%)	> 3 (%)	> 6 (%)
Cantril et al. (1974)	242	58	–	28	–
Perez et al. (1977)	81	52	–	22	–
Harisiadis et al. (1978)	146	–	70	–	32

only 32% for 25 patients in whom there was a delay of more than 6 months. Perez et al. (1977) obtained a 5-year disease-free rate of 52% for 31 patients with B1 and C disease treated promptly with radiotherapy, compared with only 22% for 18 patients who had a delay to treatment of 3–12 months. Cantril et al. (1974) found local failure following radiotherapy in 12% of 198 patients with a treatment delay of up to 3 months, in contrast to 30% for 44 patients with a delay of 4 months or more.

In relation to the concept of tumour latency and deferred treatment for incidental focal prostatic tumours, it is important to distinguish between well-defined, well-differentiated neoplasms (A1) and the more diffuse, poorly-differentiated lesions (A2). The former may be watched with little risk, whilst the latter should be treated promptly and aggressively. Similarly, for categories T1 and T2 the small asymptomatic well-differentiated nodule must be distinguished from the more extensive and generally less well-differentiated lesion. Here again, the former may be watched whilst the latter should be treated without delay.

8 Other Approaches to Treatment

8.1 Improved Radiation Schedules

Apart from modifying dose-time-volume factors in radiotherapy to avoid sequelae, there is a possibility of developing a more effective treatment schedule based, principally, on changes in irradiation fractionation. The aim of such changes would be to increase the tumour-lethal effect whilst improving the therapeutic ratio. There have been few observations concerning this aspect of prostatic cancer therapy. In a randomized study Lloyd-Davis et al. (1971) found that treatment with six fractions of irradiation over 18 days to deliver a total tumour dose of 3,750 rads was producing, in the early stages of the trial, a survival pattern no better than that following treatment with stilboestrol.

8.2 Combined Irradiation and Endocrine Treatment

Scott and Boyd (1969) used endocrine methods of treatment (castration or oestrogen administration) in patients with limited extraprostatic spread in an attempt to render

Table 16. Failure of oestrogen therapy to improve results of irradiation in patients with stage C carcinoma of prostate. Results of randomized trial at M. D. Anderson Hospital. (Actuarial survival rates read from graphs.) Neglia et al. (1977)

Treatment	Patients	Local control (%)	5-Year survival (%)
RT	40	90	73
RT + oestrogen	38	87	60

such cases technically more suitable for major surgery. Radical prostatectomy was performed after an interval of 6 months in those patients showing a response to the preliminary endocrine treatment. The 5- and 10-year disease-free survival rates following the combined treatment were 61% (24/44) and 51% (17/33), respectively. These results are comparable to those of radical operation alone reported by Jewett (1969) for patients with early tumours histologically confined to the prostate. Preliminary endocrine treatment may therefore prepare the ground for possible cure, or at least long-term control, by surgery in patients with moderately advanced diseases. Is there a role for endocrine treatment prior to or with radiotherapy? Although one may be encouraged by the experience of Scott and Boyd (1969), the Stanford group found no significant difference between patients receiving or not receiving pre-irradiation hormone treatment (Ray and Bagshaw 1975). At present, there is no evidence that endocrine therapy can improve the results of radiotherapy. On the contrary, inferior results have been reported with regard to both local tumour control and patient survival following castration or oestrogen administration prior to or concomitant with radiotherapy, compared with radiotherapy alone (Cantril et al. 1974; de Muelenaere and Sandison 1976; Werf-Messing et al. 1976; Cox and Stoffel 1977; Perez et al. 1977; Neglia et al. 1977; Taylor et al. 1979). For example, de Muelenaere and Sandison (1976) found a local recurrence rate of 32% among 19 patients treated by radiotherapy and oestrogen, compared with only 10% in 20 patients receiving radiotherapy alone. Neglia et al. (1977), in both historical and randomized studies, found no increase in local tumour control or in survival rates for a combination of radiotherapy and oestrogen (1–5 mg daily) compared with radiotherapy alone (Table 16). The increased mortality in patients receiving adjuvant oestrogen therapy is probably due to cardiovascular complications. De Muelenaere and Sandison (1976) reported thrombo-embolic deaths in 29% of 34 patients receiving oestrogen in addition to radiotherapy, compared with only 3% among 32 patients treated by radiotherapy alone.

It is possible that in patients with bulky primary or/and nodal disease a planned *short* course of oestrogen therapy or, alternatively, castration prior to extended-volume radiotherapy may reduce tumour mass and permit at least more rapid control of the disease. Such endocrine measures, especially castration, as a preliminary to radiotherapy have been of value in reducing ureteric obstruction (Michigan and Catalona 1977). Green et al. (1979) reported good responses in patients with gross nodal disease following a combination of oestrogen and extended-volume irradiation; 17 of 25 (68%) such patients remained disease-free for 1.5–7 years.

From the available evidence it must be concluded that in general, combined treatment with radiotherapy and endocrine manipulation, principally oestrogen administration, does not increase the effect of irradiation against prostatic cancer. Local tumour response is not increased by the concomitant oestrogen, and survival may in fact be reduced because of the increased incidence of thrombo-embolic deaths.

8.3 Postoperative Radiotherapy

Several authors have referred to the value of postoperative irradiation in patients with residual or recurrent prostatic tumour following radical surgery (Cantril et al. 1974; Ray et al. 1975; Taylor 1977; Neglia et al. 1977). Ray et al. (1975) reported eight of 21 such cases alive without evidence of disease 2–8 years after 'salvage' irradiation.

8.4 Preoperative Radiotherapy

Perhaps preoperative irradiation, as in patients with locally advanced bladder cancer (Wallace and Bloom 1976; Whitmore et al. 1977), may hold some promise for selected patients with carcinoma of the prostate, especially borderline operable tumours. Preoperative extended-field irradiation has been used by Charyulu et al. (1979) with encouraging early results.

8.5 Combination of Interstitial and External Beam Therapy

The combination of interstitial and external beam therapy appears to offer the advantage of local high-dose treatment for the primary tumour and larger-volume, lower-dose treatment to try to eradicate any microscopic spread in the extraprostatic tissue and regional lymph nodes. In patients treated by implantation of iodine-125 seeds, Whitmore et al. (1979) gave supplementary external beam irradiation to the pelvis and, in some patients with histologically positive pelvic nodes, to the para-aortic region: preliminary observations suggest that this additional treatment may be of benefit.

Chan and Gutierrez (1976) used a combination of a gold-198 grain implant and strictly localised external beam irradiation to achieve a more uniform high-dose treatment for the primary tumour in patients with limited extraprostatic spread. The aim was to deliver an implant dose of 4,000 rads plus an additional 4,000 rads from cobalt-60 irradiation: no results were reported.

Carlton and his colleagues (Carlton et al. 1975; Guerriero et al. 1979) employed a combination of gold-198 grains (to give a dose of 3,000–3,500 rads), external beam therapy over very small fields of 4 × 4 cm (to deliver 4,000–4,500 rads), and lymphadenectomy. The preliminary 5-year survival rates for the surgically staged node-free patients were encouraging, but longer-term observations are required.

8.6 Reduction of Radioresistance of Hypoxic Tumour Cells

The presence of hypoxic malignant cells resulting from tumour growth outstripping its blood supply is generally considered to be the principal underlying cause of tumour radio-resistance. It is assumed that such hypoxic but viable clonogenic cells remaining in a tumour after radiotherapy act as foci for recurrence. Physical methods of trying to overcome tissue hypoxia for cancer therapy, such as breathing oxygen under pressure, have now been largely superseded by chemical methods.

Extensive laboratory and clinical research is being undertaken to find chemicals capable of increasing cell radiosensitivity. Attention is focussed principally on electron-affinic compounds, chiefly the derivatives of nitroimidazole, such as metronidazole and misonidazole (see review by Adams 1977). These agents, like oxygen, selectively sensitize hypoxic cells to irradiation in all phases of the cell cycle and, not being rapidly metabolised like oxygen, are expected to penetrate deeply beyond the capillarie into the central hypoxic zones of the tumour.

There is evidence that the nitroimidazole drugs may also possess a selective direct cytotoxic action against hypoxic cells. Thus, we now have the possibility of advancing treatment with agents possessing both radiosensitising and cytotoxic properties. Results of various controlled clinical cancer trials are awaited with interest. Prostatic cancer would seem to be an eminently suitable tumour for such a study. The administration of misonidazole during irradiation may help to eradicate those residual tumour cells found in prostatic biopsies some months after radiotherapy, the presence of which is raising doubts as to the value of radiotherapy in such cases.

High LET irradiation such as fast neutrons is less dependent on the presence of oxygen or on the phase of the cell cycle than X- or gamma-rays for its biological effects. On the basis of in vitro and in vivo studies, neutron therapy is expected to be some 20%–30% more effective than X-rays. Reports from the Medical Research Council's Cyclotron Unit at Hammersmith Hospital, where more than 800 patients with various tumours have been treated with 7.5 MeV neutrons, suggest that with such treatment a greater degree of local control is achieved compared with X-rays, especially in certain tumours considered to be relatively radio-resistant to conventional treatment. It seems that bulky, localised prostatic cancer would be a good example for a trial of neutron irradiation but, so far, no such experience has been reported.

8.7 Adjuvant Chemotherapy

A wide variety of cytotoxic agents, singly or in combination, have been tried in patients with advanced hormone-resistant cancer of the prostate, but with no impressive or consistent success. A trial of cytotoxic agents in patients with advanced prostatic cancer is often hampered by impaired renal function and also a reduced marrow reserve resulting from tumour infiltration and previous irradiation.

Objective responses in patients with advanced prostatic cancer have been reported following treatment with certain single agents, principally 5-fluorouracil, nitrogen mustard, cyclophosphamide, and hydroxyurea. A number of trials with these and other drugs are in progress. When active single agents have been discovered and their combination shown to be effective in patients with disseminated cancer then their use as adjuvants in the primary management of the disease will be explored. Preliminary observations in our urology unit with methotrexate alone or in combination with cytoxan or with cytoxan and 5-fluorouracil in hormone-resistant cases have been encouraging: objective responses were seen in six of 17 patients (35%) (Jones and Williams 1980). Similar response rates have been reported recently by Ihde et al. (1980) for adriamycin plus cytoxan (32%) and by Franks (1979) for melphalan (33%).

9 Conclusions

Until some 15 years ago radiotherapy was generally regarded as an occasional palliative treatment for cancer of the prostate, to be used mainly against painful skeletal metastases in hormone-resistant cases. Its application in this disease has now become much wider, with the prospect of achieving long-term control or even cure in patients with early or even locally advanced disease, without the complications associated with surgery and the side-effects of endocrine treatment.

At present, the most appropriate treatment for primary prostatic cancer should be selected after taking into account tumour stage and grade, the age and general condition of the patient, any previous treatment, the available facilities, and not least, the effective procedure which interferes least with quality of life.

Non-palpable, focal, well-differentiated tumours found in surgical specimens (T0) or forming a small clinical nodule (T1) may be treated expectantly in the first instance to assess whether the tumour is active or not. More diffuse and less well-differentiated focal or localised tumours (T0–T2) should be treated aggressively from the outset, especially in younger patients, and for such cases either radical prostatectomy or interstitial irradiation would apparently be appropriate.

Interstitial irradiation, with its low morbidity, appears to provide a serious challenge to radical surgery in the curative treatment of early cases. However, information regarding involvement of lymph nodes removed at the time of implant reveals that many apparently early tumours clinically confined to the prostate are, in fact, advanced due to regional lymph node spread. In such cases it seems that external beam irradiation from the outset, or as a supplement to interstitial irradiation, would be more suitable.

Tumours with clinical extension into the periprostatic tissues should also be treated with the aim of cure or long-term control. It is in this group that regional nodes are more likely to be involved but, hopefully, only to a limited extent. Large-field external beam therapy to encompass the pelvic nodes and, in some patients, the para-aortic region seems to be the most appropriate treatment for such cases. In patients with more advanced extraprostatic spread, often with substantial node involvement, treatment should be by external beam irradiation, but the results are likely to be only palliative.

The value of radiotherapy in primary cases of prostatic cancer must be judged not only by survival rates, but also by its ability to control local disease and thereby spare the patient the distress of advancing pelvic malignancy. Reported experience shows that pelvic irradiation can effectively control local disease in some 90% of patients. The morbidity of radical external beam radiotherapy is low, but there appears to be a surprisingly high incidence of impotence and this requires further evaluation.

Endocrine manipulation, which can only be of temporary value and, in the case of oestrogen administration, carries an increased mortality due to cardiovascular complications, should not be used in the primary treatment of local-regional disease, but held in reserve for radiotherapy failures. So far, the majority of reports fail to show that concomitent or prior endocrine treatment improves radiotherapy results.

In most reports concerning radiotherapy for patients with prostatic cancer the period of follow-up rarely exceeds 5 years. Although the preliminary survival rates are encouraging, the natural history of this disease calls for longer-term results before the role of interstitial or/and external beam techniques can be adequately assessed.

10 References

Adams GE (1977) Hypoxic cell sensitizers for radiotherapy. In: Becker FF (ed) Cancer: a comprehensive treatise, vol 6. Plenum Press, New York London, pp 181–223
Bagshaw MA (1978) Radiation therapy for carcinoma of the prostate. In: Skinner DG, de Kernion JB (eds) Genitourinary cancer. Saunders, Philadelphia London, pp 355–379
Bagshaw MA, Kaplan HS, Sagerman RH (1965) Linear accelerator supervoltage radiotherapy. VII. Carcinoma of the prostate. Radiology 85: 121–129
Bloom HJG, Hendry WF (1973) Treatment of prostatic cancer. In: Raven RW (ed) Modern trends in oncology, part 2. Butterworths, London, pp 143–180
Budhraja SN, Anderson JC (1964) An assessment of the value of radiotherapy in the management of carcinoma of the prostate. Br J Urol 36: 535–540
Cantril ST, Vaeth JM, Green JP, Schroeder AF (1974) Radiation therapy for localized carcinoma of the prostate: Correlation with histopathological grading. Frontiers of Radiation Therapy and Oncology 9: 274–294
Carlton CE, Hudgins PT, Guerriero WG, Scott R (1975) Radiotherapy in the management of stage C carcinoma of the prostate. Trans Am Assoc Genitourin Surg 67: 70–74
Cerny JC, Farah R, Rian R, Weckstein ML (1975) An evaluation of lymphangiography in staging carcinoma of the prostate. J Urol 113: 367–370
Chan RC, Gutierrez AE (1976) Carcinoma of the prostate: its treatment by a combination of radioactive gold grain implant and external irradiation. Cancer 37: 2749–2754
Charyulu K, Block N, Sudarsanam A (1979) Preoperative extended field radiation with I 125 seed implant in prostatic cancer: a preliminary report for a randomized study. Int J Radiat Oncol Biol Phys 5: 1957–1961
Cosgrove MD, Kaempf MJ (1976) Prostatic cancer revisited. J Urol 115: 79–81
Court B, Chassagne D (1977) Interstitial radiation therapy of cancer of the prostate using iridium-192 wires. Cancer Treat Rep 61: 329–330
Cox JD, Stoffel TJ (1977) The significance of needle biopsy after irradiation for stage C adenocarcinoma of the prostate. Cancer 40: 156–160
Dahl DS, Wilson CS, Middleton RG, Bourne HH (1974) Pelvic lymphadenectomy for staging localized prostatic cancer. J Urol 112: 245–246
De Muelenaere GFGO, Sandison AG (1976) Treatment of locally advanced prostatic carcinoma. Br J Radiol 49: 944–947
Del Regato JA (1967) Radiotherapy in the conservative treatment of operable and locally inoperable carcinoma of the prostate. Radiology 88: 761–766
Donohue RE, Fauver HE, Whitesel JA, Pfister RR (1979) Staging prostatic cancer: a different distribution. J Urol 122: 327–329
Franks CR (1979) Melphelan in metastatic cancer of the prostate. Cancer Treat Rev [Suppl] 6: 121–125
Flocks RH (1969) Present status of interstitial irradiation in managing prostatic cancer. JAMA 210: 328–330
Flocks RH, Kerr HD, Elkins HB, Culp D (1952) Treatment of carcinoma of the prostate by interstitial radiation with radioactive gold Au-198: a preliminary report. J Urol 68: 510–522
George FW, Carlton CE, Dykhuizen RF, Dillon JR (1965) Cobalt-60 telecurietherapy in the definitive treatment of carcinoma of the prostate: a preliminary report. J Urol 93:102–109
Golimbu M, Morales P, Al-Askari S, Brown J (1979) Extended pelvic lymphadenectomy for prostatic cancer. J Urol 121: 617–620
Green N, Melbye RW, Iba G (1978) Radiation therapy for carcinoma of the prostate: the experience with small intestine injury. Int J Radiat Oncol Biol Phys 4: 1049–1053
Green N, Broth E, George FW, Goldstein A, Melbye RW, Morrow J, Onofrio R, Polse S, Skaist L (1979) Prostate carcinoma: therapeutic considerations in the management of gross lymph node metastases. Int J Radiat Oncol Biol Phys 5: 891–897

Guerriero WG, Barrett MT, Bartholomew T, Carlton CE, Hudgins PT (1979) Combined interstitial and external radiotherapy in the definitive management of carcinoma of the prostate. In: Johnson DE, Samuels ML (eds) Cancer of the genitourinary tract. Raven Press, New York, pp 207–216

Harisiadis L, Veenema RJ, Senyszyn JJ, Puchner PJ, Tretter P, Roma NA, Chang CH, Lattimer JK, Tannenbaum M (1978) Carcinoma of the prostate: treatment with external radiotherapy. Cancer 41:2131–2142

Herr HW (1979) Preservation of sexual potency in prostatic cancer patients after pelvic lymphadenectomy and retropubic I 125 implantation J Urol 121:621–623

Hilaris BS, Whitmore WF, Batata M, Barzell W (1977) Behavioural patterns of prostatic adenocarcinoma following an I-125 implant and pelvic node dissection. Int J Radiat Oncol Biol Phys 2:631–637

Hill DR, Crews QE, Walsh PC (1974) Prostate carcinoma: radiation treatment of the primary and regional lymphatics. Cancer 34:156–160

Howe GE, Prentiss RJ, Mullenix RB, Freeney MJ (1963) Treatment of carcinoma of the prostate with radioactive gold: nine-year follow-up. J Urol 89:73–74

Hussey DH (1979) Experience with limited field irradiation for adenocarcinoma of the prostate. In: Johnson DE, Samuels ML (eds) Cancer of the genitourinary tract. Raven Press, New York, pp 217–228

Ihde DC, Bunn PA, Cohen MH, Dunnick NR, Eddy JL, Minna JD (1980) Effective treatment of hormonally-unresponsive metastatic carcinoma of the prostate with adriamycin and cyclophosphamide. Cancer 45:1300–1310

Jewett HJ (1969) The results of radical perineal prostatectomy JAMA 210:324–325

Jones MA, Williams G (1980) The non-hormone chemotherapy of prostatic cancer. Br J Urol 52:127–130

Koehler PR (1976) Current status of lymphography in patients with cancer. Cancer 37:503–516

Lipsett JA, Cosgrove MD, Green N, Casagrande JT, Melbye RW, George FW (1976) Factors influencing prognosis in the radiotherapeutic management of carcinoma of the prostate. Int J Radiat Oncol Biol Phys 1:1049–1058

Lloyd-Davies RW, Vinnicombe J, Collins CD (1971) The treatment of localised prostatic carcinoma. Clin Radiol 32:230–234

Loh ES, Brown HE, Beiler DD (1971) Radiotherapy of carcinoma of the prostate: a preliminary report. J Urol 106:906–909

McCullough DL, Prout GR, Daly JJ (1974) Carcinoma of the prostate and lymphatic metastases. J Urol 111:65–71

McGowan DG (1977) Radiation therapy in the management of localized carcinoma of the prostate: a preliminary report. Cancer 39:98–103

McLaughlin AP, Saltzstein SL, McCullough DL, Gittes RF (1976) Prostatic carcinoma: incidence and location of unsuspected lymphatic metastases. J Urol 115:89–94

Michigan S, Catalona WJ (1977) Ureteral obstruction from prostatic carcinoma: response to endocrine and radiation therapy. J Urol 118:733–738

Nachtsheim DA, McAninch JW, Stutzman RE, Goebel JL (1978) Latent residual tumour following external radiotherapy for prostate adenocarcinoma. J Urol 120:312–314

Neglia WJ, Hussey DH, Johnson DE (1977) Megavoltage radiation therapy for carcinoma of the prostate. Int J Radiat Oncol Biol Phys 2:873–882

Odell RW, Merill MD, Atwood CJ (1971) Cobalt-60 teletherapy of localized prostatic cancer: a 10-year experience. J Urol 105:843–846

O'Donoghue EPN, Shridhar P, Sherwood T, Williams JP, Chisholm GD (1976) Lymphography and pelvic lymphadenectomy in carcinoma of the prostate. Br J Urol 48:689–696

Paxton RM, Williams G, Macdonald JS (1975) Role of lymphography in carcinoma of the prostate. Br Med J 1:120–122

Perez CA, Bauer W, Garza R, Royce RK (1977) Radiation therapy in the definitive treatment of localized carcinoma of the prostate. Cancer 40:1425–1433

Pistenma DA, Bagshaw MA, Freiha FS (1979) Extended field radiation therapy for prostatic adenocarcinoma: status report of a limited prospective trial. In: Johnson DE, Samuels ML (eds) Cancer of the genitourinary tract. Raven Press, New York, pp 229–247
Pistenma DA, Ray GR, Bagshaw MA (1976) The role of megavoltage radiation therapy in the treatment of prostatic carcinoma. Semin Oncol 3: 115–122
Ray GR, Bagshaw MA (1975) The role of radiation therapy in the definitive treatment of adenocarcinoma of the prostate. Annu Rev Med 26: 567–588
Ray GR, Cassady JR, Bagshaw MA (1973) Definitive radiation therapy of carcinoma of the prostate. Radiology 106: 407–418
Ray GR, Cassady JR, Bagshaw MA (1975) External beam megavoltage radiation therapy in the treatment of post-radical prostatectomy residual or recurrent tumour: preliminary results. J Urol 114: 98–101
Rhamy RK, Wilson SK, Caldwell WL (1972) Biopsy proved tumour following definite irradiation for resectable carcinoma of the prostate. J Urol 107: 627–630
Rubin P (1969) Supervoltage radiation therapy: promise versus fulfillment. JAMA 210: 333–335
Scott WW, Boyd HL (1969) Combined hormone control therapy and radical prostatectomy in the treatment of selected cases of advanced carcinoma of the prostate: a retrospective study based on 25 years experience. J Urol 101: 86–92
Spellman MC, Castellino RA, Ray GR, Pistenma DA, Bagshaw MA (1977) An evaluation of lymphography in localized carcinoma of the prostate. Radiology 125: 637–644
Taylor WJ (1977) Radiation oncology: cancer of the prostate. Cancer 39: 856–861
Taylor WJ, Richardson RG, Hafermann MD (1979) Radiation therapy for localized prostate cancer. Cancer 43: 1123–1127
Wallace DM, Bloom HJG (1976) The management of deeply infiltrating (T3) bladder carcinoma: controlled trial of radical radiotherapy versus pre-operative radiotherapy and radical cystectomy (first report). Br J Urol 48: 587–594
Werf-Messing B van der, Sourek-Zikova V, Blonk DI (1976) Localized advanced carcinoma of the prostate: radiation therapy versus hormonal therapy. Int J Radiat Oncol Biol Phys 1: 1043–1048
Whitmore WF, Batata M, Hilaris B (1979) Prostatic irradiation: I-125 implantation. In: Johnson DE, Samuels ML (eds) Cancer of the genitourinary tract. Raven Press, New York, pp 195–205
Whitmore WF, Hilaris BS, Grabstald H (1972) Retropubic implantation of iodine-125 in the treatment of prostatic cancer. J Urol 108: 918–920
Whitmore WF, Batata MA, Hilaris BS, Reddy GN, Unal A, Ghoneim MA, Grabstald H, Chu F (1977) A comparative study of two preoperative radiation regimens with cystectomy for bladder cancer. Cancer 40: 1077–1086

Endocrine and Cytotoxic Therapy

P. H. Smith*

Department of Urology, St. James's University Hospital, GB – Leeds

1 Introduction

A disease common enough to account for 6% of all malignant disease in the male inevitably merits serious consideration and committed research programmes. The full impact of prostatic cancer is to some extent reduced for three reasons: the diagnosis is made in over 50% of patients after the age of 65; there is a known incidence of 20%–50% of latent cancer (Wynder et al. 1971); and approximately two-thirds of patients die of some other condition (Byar 1973).

For the last 40 years treatment of prostatic cancer has been dominated by the observation of Huggins and Hodges (1941) that orchidectomy or diethylstilboestrol (DES) 1 mg/day inhibited disseminated disease. The value of oestrogen therapy with DES in doses of 1–150 mg/day was not questioned until the Veterans Administration Cooperative Research Group (VACURG) decided in 1960 to evaluate the effect of placebo, oestrogens, orchidectomy, and oestrogens plus orchidectomy on a prospective randomised basis in patients with carcinoma extending beyond the prostate gland and in those with metastatic disease. The results of this first VACURG study (1967) opened a new era by emphasising the cardiovascular toxicity of the regimes involving oestrogen therapy in the dose used – DES 5 mg/day.

Since 1967 there has been great interest in the management of this disease, with particular emphasis being placed upon the indications for oestrogen therapy, the development of alternative treatments including other hormonal agents, the possible value of radiotherapy and radical surgery, and the concept of deferring treatment until merited by symptoms of metastatic disease.

In their second, third, and focal studies VACURG have contributed information on the further evaluation of DES and of alternative hormonal agents (Byar 1973, 1980). The seond VACURG study compared DES at doses of 0.2, 1.0, and 5 mg/day for those with disease clinically beyond the prostatic capsule. In the third VACURG study DES 1 mg/day was compared with Provera 30 mg/day, Provera 30 mg + DES 1 mg/day, and Premarin 2.5 mg/day in patients in these same stages of disease. This group also evaluated the role of radical prostatectomy with or without additional oestrogen therapy in the first study and radical prostatectomy against placebo in the second and third studies, in patients with coincidentally discovered disease and in patients with malignant nodules clinically localised within the prostate. In the focal study patients

* I should like to acknowledge my thanks to Miss S. A. Barrowby for her help in the preparation of this paper

© Springer-Verlag Berlin · Heidelberg 1981

Table 1. Outline of the protocols of the National Prostatic Cancer Project

Metastatic disease					
Failed on conventional treatment					
No. 100	Cyclophosphamide	vs	5-fluorouracil	vs	'standard'
No. 300	Cyclophosphamide	vs	DTIC	vs	procarbazine
No. 700	Cyclophosphamide	vs	methyl-CCNU	vs	hydroxyurea
Failed on conventional treatment + more than 2,000 rad to pelvis					
No. 200	Estracyt	vs	streptozotocin	vs	'standard'
No. 400	Prednimustine	vs	Estracyt + prednimustine		
No. 800	Estracyt	vs	vincristine	vs	Estracyt + vincristine
Newly diagnosed					
No. 500	DES or orchidectomy	vs	DES + cyclophosphamide	vs	Estracyt + cyclophosphamide
Stable with hormone therapy					
No. 600	DES	vs	DES + cyclophosphamide	vs	Estracyt + DES
Localized disease					
After radical prostatectomy					
No. 900	No additional treatment	vs	cyclophosphamide	vs	Estracyt
After radical radiotherapy					
No. 1000	No additional treatment	vs	cyclophosphamide	vs	Estracyt

Table 2. Outline of eortic protocols for patients with prostatic cancer

Patients with advanced disease (T3–4, M0; T0–4, M1)			
Protocol 30761			
DES 1 mg t.d.s. vs	Cyproterone acetate 250 mg/day PO	vs	Medroxyprogesterone acetate 500 mg IM three times weekly for 2 months then 100 mg PO b.d.
Protocol 30762			
DES 1 mg t.d.s. vs	Estracyt 280 mg b.d. for 8 weeks and 140 mg b.d. thereafter		
Patients with advanced disease who have failed on conventional treatment			
Protocol 30763 – Comparative phase II study			
Adriamycin 60 mg/m^2 every 3 weeks	vs	Procarbazine 200 mg/day on days 1–14 of each 28-day cycle	
Protocol 30799 – Phase II study			
Vindesine 3 mg/m^2 weekly, increasing by 0.5 mg/m^2 (subject to toxicity) to a maximum of 4 mg/m^2			

with coincidentally discovered disease who were too old or too ill, or who refused radical prostatectomy were treated by the same regimen as was used for those with advanced disease in study 1. The results of these studies are considered under the section on hormonal therapy.
In 1972 the National Prostatic Cancer Project (NPCP) was formed and made the first concerted effort to investigate the potential of cytotoxic chemotherapy in patients with prostatic cancer. The NPCP has now implemented ten different protocols for the assessment of different treatment regimes (Beckley et al. 1979), in addition to undertaking a large programme of scientific research. An outline of these studies is shown in Table 1.
In 1976 the European Organisation for Research on the Treatment of Cancer (EORTC) brought together two existing clinical research groups to form the EORTC Urological Group, which has since implemented four protocols for the investigation of hormonal and chemotherapy. A brief outline of these studies is shown in Table 2.

2 Clinical Classification of Prostatic Cancer

During the last 20 years three major systems of clinical classification have been used – the VACURG system, that recommeneded by the American Urological Association (AUA), and that of the Union International contre le Cancer, i.e., the TNM system (see this volume, Chap. 9). To minimise confusion and to allow comparison of the results of the different studies the systems are compared in Table 3. In this chapter the VACURG system will be used when considering the conclusions of the Veterans Administration, the AUA system adopted by the NPCP when the studies organised by that body are assessed, and the TNM system used by the EORTC group, when dealing with EORTC protocols.

Table 3. Comparison of staging systems proposed by VACURG, UICC (TNM system), and AUA

VACURG	TNM		AUA	Rectal examination
I	M0	T0	A	
II		T1–2	B	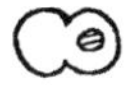
III		T3–4	C	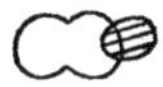
IV	M1	T0–4	D	Any of above

3 Hormone Therapy

3.1 Contribution of the Veterans Administration Cooperative Research Group

The three main Veterans Administration studies have now been analysed on several occasions and, together with several smaller studies, present a complex and almost overwhelming amount of information. It is best to consider this information under the headings of the different stages of the disease.

Stage I Disease (Coincidentally Diagnosed Cancer). The incidence of coincidentally diagnosed disease in the first VACURG study was 5.75% of the total. Treatment was designed to assess the value of oestrogen therapy following radical prostatectomy. In the second and third studies the comparison was between radical prostatectomy and placebo.

Survival figures for these studies have recently been published (Byar 1980), and show no evidence that radical prostatectomy with or without oestrogen therapy is superior to placebo treatment. The fact that certain patients developed disseminated disease despite radical surgery for clinically localised lesions casts very grave doubt upon the advisability of such an approach, and questions even the use of radiotherapy in this situation, which though infinitely less traumatic, is still not without some morbidity. It also reinforces the concept of micrometastatic tumors and supports the exploration of the role of cytotoxic chemotherapy in patients with such early lesions.

During the period of recruitment to these studies several patients did not undergo prostatectomy as they were too old or too ill or refused radical prostatectomy. These patients were entered into the focal study, in which they were treated just as the patients with stage III and stage IV disease in the first study. The results of this study (Byar et al. 1972) showed no evidence of superiority of treatment over placebo, and Byar noted that only 6.8% of patients showed progression, whilst no patient died of prostatic cancer. The combined figures for this study and four others quoted showed only five deaths from prostatic cancer in 262 patients (1.9%).

Table 4. Incidence of death from prostatic cancer in patients with stage I disease

	Patients	Died of prostatic cancer
Correa et al. (1974)	47	2
Byar (1972) (combined statistics)	262	5
Blackard et al. (1971)	91	2
Total	400	9 (2.25%)

Since that report emphasis has been placed upon the concept of 'diffuse' and 'focal' stage I disease. Correa et al. (1974) studied 47 stage I patients, eight of whom had diffuse and 39 focal disease. Treatment was DES 1 mg/day (23 patients), radical prostatectomy (2 patients) and no therapy (22 patients). Diffuse carcinoma was found in eight patients, five of whom (62%) showed progression of tumor with two deaths. Only three of the 39 patients with focal disease experienced progression, and none died of prostatic cancer. Treatment was evenly distributed within the two groups, except that both patients undergoing radical prostatectomy had focal disease. These authors believe that treatment in both groups should be delayed until clinically detectable disease appears, since with either treatment survival is very similar to that of the normal male population of a similar age. It may, however, be more logical to treat all patients with diffuse disease in view of the known high rate of progression.

The combined figures from this study, the results reported in the paper by Byar et al. (1972), and those of Blackard et al. (1971) are shown in Table 4.

These findings are of increasing importance since more patients are now being diagnosed at an early stage of the disease, 37% of patients presenting with stage I disease in a recent study by Donohue et al. (1979).

Stage II Disease (Localised Nodule Within Normal Prostate). Patients with nodular lesions were treated in the same way as those with Stage I disease and the results reported by Byar (1980) are broadly similar but do demonstrate a reduction in the progression rate ($p = 0.025$) with oestrogen therapy combined with radical operation. However, the differences in progression rates compared with a smaller group of patients treated by radical operation or placebo were not significant. Moreover, the survival figures in both groups are virtually identical – again questioning the value of radical operation and demonstrating that very few patients with stage I or stage II disease die of prostatic cancer (6 of 150 patients with stage I and 11 of 208 patients with stage II disease).

Stage III Disease (Disease Extending beyond the Prostatic Capsule). Tumours classed as stage III disease are obviously active rather than latent, and it is now recognised that in 40%–50% of cases there are already metastases in the lymph nodes. Despite this, progression is slow, only 50% of patients developing clinical metastases within 4 years even when initially treated with placebo. Orchidectomy or the administration of hormones delays progression (Byar 1973) but does not affect the overall survival of the patient, because of an excess of cardiovascular deaths in those receiving hormones and an excess of deaths from cardiovascular and other causes in those treated by orchidectomy (Jordan et al. 1977).

Stage IV Disease (Evidence of Metastases). In patients with stage IV disease, the first study showed that oestrogen therapy was not associated with undue cardiovascular hazard and that although oestrogen therapy and orchidectomy relieved symptoms of metastases no increase in survival was seen when compared with placebo as initial therapy. The combination of oestrogen and orchidectomy was not superior to either alone and there was no evidence that orchidectomy was superior to oestrogens.
The disappointing nature of these results, the emphasis on the cardiovascular toxicity of DES 5 mg/day, the realisation that radical surgery neither increases survival nor prevents the development of metastatic disease, and the recognition that the effect of hormonal therapy is largely palliative, since its use at an early stage is not associated with increased survival, have led to the recent urgent search for alternative forms of therapy.

Second and Third VACURG Studies. In the second VACURG study in which DES doses of 0.2, 1.0, and 5.0 mg/day were compared, it was clearly demonstrated that doses of 1.0 and 5 mg/day were effective in relieving symptoms of prostatic cancer and that 1 mg/day was not associated with any cardiovascular hazard (Byar 1973). However, by this time Robinson and Thomas (1971) had shown that suppression of plasma testosterone throughout the 24 h was achieved not by DES 1 mg/day but by the dose of 1 mg t.d.s., which is now the most commonly used regimen even though its cardiovascular hazard, if any, is still unknown.
In the third study VACURG started the search for alternative compounds by comparing the effects of DES 1 mg daily against those of Premarin 2.5 mg/day, Provera 30 mg/day, and Provera 30 mg/day plus DES 1 mg/day. None of these regimens showed any advantage over DES (Byar 1980).

Reconsideration of VACURG Studies. In evaluating the VACURG studies it is important to remember that (a) the concept of diffuse and focal stage I disease has appeared since the VACURG studies were designed; (b) the studies took no account of predisposition to cardiovascular complications. If the same study was repeated after excluding patients with pre-existing cardiovascular disease a different result might be obtained, especially in patients with stage III and IV disease; and (c) no randomised study comparing DES 1 mg/day with other agents has yet been published.

3.2 Alternative Hormone Therapy

Ever since the introduction of oestrogen therapy and orchidectomy it has been recognised that some patients do not respond, whilst others develop signs and symptoms of progression after a period of satisfactory control. The possible roles of adrenalectomy and hypophysectomy were considered at an early stage, but although relief of bone pain may be dramatic, the remission of symptoms is often of short duration (Silverberg 1977).
Alternative drug therapy may involve the use of other oestrogens, progestogens, anti-androgens, and medical adrenalectomy in the desire to suppress or abolish androgen stimulation of the prostatic cells.
The known physiological actions of these different agents are well reviewed by Menon and Walsh (1979) and are briefly summarised in Table 5. These authors confirm that orchidectomy causes a sustained suppression of plasma testosterone and note that the

use of adrenalectomy and hyphophysectomy, though helpful in certain patients, is somewhat illogical since adult prepubertal castrates all have atrophic prostates with no secretion.

Although many people in the United Kingdom still accept DES as the first choice for hormonal therapy, others have a strong feeling that orchidectomy is preferable. This controversy, together with the true objective remission rates of each therapy and the cardiovascular hazard if any of DES 1 mg t.d.s. remains to be resolved.

Alternative oestrogens, progestogens, anti-androgens, and Estracyt (combining oestrogens with a cytotoxic agent) have been used for some years, usually to treat

Table 5. Summary of major actions of oestrogens, progestogens and anti-androgens. After Menon and Walsh (1979)

	Oestrogens	Progestogens	Anti-androgens
Gonadotrophin secretion	↓	↓	↓
Production of testosterone	↓	↓	↓
Conversion of testosterone to dihydrotestosterone (DHT)	↓		↓
Binding of DHT by prostatic nuclei		↓	↓

Table 6. Agents of potential value in the treatment of cancer of the prostate (remissions/evaluable patients)[a]

Aminoglutethimide	15/28
Cyproterone acetate	71/117
Depostat	0/5
Estracyt	208/528
Flutamide	20/43
Honvan	95/161
Megestrol acetate	12/13
Tace	6/14

[a] By kind permission of S. Karger AG

Table 7. Costs of hormonal agents for the treatment of prostatic cancer (United Kingdom, February 1980)

	Cost/tablet	
	Actual	Relative[a]
DES, 1 mg	0.3 p	1
Ethinyl estradiol, 1 mg	0.8 p	3
Tace, 12 mg	3.5 p	12
Honvan, 100 mg	6.4 p	21
Medroxyprogesterone acetate, 100 mg	34.8 p	116
Cyproterone acetate, 50 mg	66.0 p	220
Estracyt, 140 mg	107.0 p	356

[a] To nearest whole number

patients who have failed on conventional hormone therapy. The literature, though not extensive, is difficult to interpret, as the subjective relief experienced is not necessarily associated with objective remission, and the true value of these agents in both newly diagnosed and relapsed patients remains to be established. The subject has recently been reviewed (Smith 1980), and the incidence of response and the costs of these alternative agents are shown in Tables 6 and 7. The challenge of the 1970s has been to obtain further information on alternative forms of therapy by means of prospective randomised clinical trials.

4 The Use of Clinical Trials in Prostatic Cancer

Despite the example of the VACURG many people are still uncertain of the rules governing clinical trials, unaware of the complexity of the necessary administrative machinery, and doubtful of their necessity. It is therefore desirable to review some of the basic concepts.

All medical progress is dependent upon the generation of new ideas which, when tested by individuals or small groups, offer some hope of progress. At this stage the concept has to be evaluated in an orderly manner by means of a recognised pattern of trials, each of increasing complexity. These are outlined below.

4.1 Phase I Trials

A new agent is tested in the human to determine its maximal safe dose and to establish its toxicity. Once such a study has demonstrated the practicability of its use, its effect in a given condition is determined by a phase II trial.

4.2 Phase II Trials

The incidence of remission in the disease for which the preparation is used is evaluated. Phase II studies are usually carried out in patients with advanced disease for whom no other treatment is possible, and it is recognised that any remission may be of short duration. A remission even of short duration in such a patient, however, suggests that the agent may be of great benefit if used at an earlier stage of the disease. Such studies are of greater value if they are comparative, assessing the new agent against one for which some information is already available and which can act as a baseline. In a phase II study it is essential to continue the study until there are at lease 20–30 evaluable patients (in each arm if the study is comparative). At this point the statistician can advise on whether the study should be stopped or continued. Unless two or three objective remissions have been seen by this time it is accepted that the agent is unlikely to be of value. The evaluation of all patients showing a remission should be subjected to critical review by the study co-ordinator.

4.3 Phase III Trials

When an agent or treatment is deemed to be of value it is possible to compare it with another established form of therapy (or potentially valuable treatment from another phase II study) by means of a randomised prospective study. Whether or not the services of a professional statistician have been used for phase I and phase II studies there can be no doubt that they are essential in phase III studies. The statistician should be involved from the first, to ensure that the study is justified and that its design, implementation, monitoring, and ultimate evaluation are valid. The number of evaluable patients required in each arm varies according to the percentage remission expected in the established treatment, the percentage improvement regarded as obtainable, and the acceptable risk of missing such an improvement. In general, if one wished to discover an improvement of not less than 20% and to have only a 5% chance of failing to detect such a result, it will be necessary to have at least 100 evaluable patients in each arm. Even in experienced co-operative groups a 'non-evaluability' rate of 20%–25% is usual and one must therefore be prepared to recruit at least 125 patients to each arm. Such a trial cannot ethically be stopped until the required number of evaluable patients is available, and the commitment of the clinicians must be absolute if useful information is to emerge. Ideally such studies should only start if all are agreed that recruitment is possible within 2 years, as interest fades after that time and it is usually wise to recognise at the outset that clinicians tend to be over-optimistic in estimating the number of patients that they can enter.

For each study there must be a clearly defined protocol including an adequate introduction reviewing the literature and statements on the objectives of the trial, selection of patients, trial design, treatment, expected toxicity, investigations required before entry and at defined periods of follow-up, criteria of evaluation, instructions on registration and randomisation, statistical considerations, administrative responsibilities, references from the literature, and appropriate forms.

For such studies part-time secretarial, nursing, or medical assistance is almost essential in each active centre. To minimise the number of non-evaluable patients it is essential to have an active data centre and regular meetings of members to consider entry rates and problems with forms, and to learn of unexpected toxicity. Unless a very clear difference in treatment emerges early, one must also accept that the statistician is most unlikely to give information on the response rates of the treatments being compared until the trial is closed to recruitment.

4.4 Phase IV Trials

The adjuvant trial, in which two apparently beneficial treatments are combined and compared against one of the treatments used alone, is similar to a phase III study and equally demanding.

Although many people find this degree of commitment irksome it is otherwise impossible to compare treatments adequately, since changes in diseases, selection of patients, surgical competence, and other aspects of medical care may render the results invalid.

Those who object to controlled clinical trials observe that variations in patient entry with subsequent bias are still possible. It is prudent to admit that all systems are imperfect and that the results of any trial need to be interpreted with an open mind and with healthy scepticism. They do, however, represent an important collection of data which on re-analysis at intervals leads towards the truth.

5 The EORTC Urological Group

When the EORTC set up its Urological Group in 1976 it was made clear that the services of its extensive Data Center were available and that the Group was expected to develop suitable clinical trials. At that time the clinical interest lay in the evaluation of hormonal agents alternative to DES for the treatment of newly diagnosed advanced prostatic cancer and in contributing to the developing knowledge of cytotoxic chemotherapy in prostatic cancer. The group has implemented two protocols for each category of patients.

In considering studies for patients with newly diagnosed advanced prostatic cancer it was recognised that (a) although DES produces symptomatic relief in the majority of patients there was no evidence of the true objective remission rates; (b) the cardiovascular hazard of DES 1 mg t.d.s. was unknown; and (c) it was desirable to establish the potential value of progestogens, antiandrogens, and Estracyt in the primary treatment of advanced prostatic cancer.

Accordingly two protocols were developed to obtain certain information on these points (as previously described in Table 2).

Protocol 30761 (Co-ordinator M. Pavone-Macaluso, Palermo) had recruited 233 patients at 11 February 1980. The last evaluation was carried out in October 1979, when there were 167 evaluable patients, and the relevant findings are shown in Table 8.

Table 8. Preliminary analysis of EORTC protocol 30761, at 4 October 1979 to show reasons for patients' withdrawal from study

Treatment	Cyproterone acetate	Medroxy-progesterone acetate	Stilboestrol	Total
Progression (two deaths during MPA medication)	18 (33%)	22 (41%)	11 (19%)	51 (31%)
Excessive toxicity	1	2	2	5
Death 2 from cardiovascular causes 1 from unknown cause 1 from associated chronic disease	1 (CV)	–	3 (1CV)	4
Lost to follow-up	1	3	–	4
Treatment refused	1	1	1	3
Protocol violation	1	–	2	3
Other	3	2	–	5
Total	26/55	30/54	19/58	75/167

Table 9. Preliminary analysis of EORTC protocol 30762, at 22 October 1979 to show reasons for patients' withdrawal from study

Reason for withdrawal	Estracyt	Stilboestrol	Total
Progression (including death due to malignant disease)	23 (21%)	12 (12%)	35 (17%)
Cardiovascular death	4 (4%)	8 (8%)	12 (6%)
Excessive toxicity	5	7	12 (6%)
Treatment refused	2	2	4
Death Associated chronic disease infection	2	1	3
Lost to follow-up	–	1	1
Other	4	2	6
Total	40/107	33/97	73/204

Table 10. EORTC protocol 30762: Causes of death classed by treatment as of 22 October 1979

Cause of death	Estracyt	Stilboestrol	Total
Malignant disease	16 (15%)	11 (11%)	27 (13%)
Cardiovascular	5 (5%)	8 (8%)	13 (6%)
Associated chronic disease	3	1	4
Infection	1	–	1
Other	–	1	1
Total	25/107	21/97	46/204

These results, admittedly at an early stage in the trial, show an apparent difference between the treatment arms in terms of progression, but the patients have not yet been on study long enough to see whether there is likely to be a difference in survival.

Protocol 30762 (Co-ordinator F. Lund, Copenhagen) had recruited 310 patients at 11 February 1980. Its most recent evaluation was also carried out in October 1979, when there were 204 evaluable patients. The relevant findings are shown in Tables 9 and 10.

This study also shows a difference in progression rate between the two treatments, with some very preliminary observations on cardiovascular deaths.

Although further information on progression and survival rates will soon emerge it has become clear from the preliminary evaluations that there are several problems in determining objective remission. The evaluation criteria of complete remission, partial remission, stable disease, and progression are clearly defined in both protocols and are identical. The interpretation of the data obtained is difficult, however, and although progression is easily determined the problems of evaluation of remission merit further consideration.

6 Evaluation of Remission in Prostatic Cancer

Although it has long been recognised that prostatic cancer is often stable for long periods with or without treatment, it has been less clear until recent times that objective remission, as distinct from subjective improvement, occurs only over a prolonged time scale.

The problems concern the evaluation of T and M categories, since (a) the T category is assessed by rectal palpation and is subject to observer variation, and (b) the M category is usually associated with deposits in bones, which resolve slowly if at all. The assessment of bone metastases by X-ray is complicated by the necessity of deciding whether increasing sclerosis represents healing or progression. Assessment by scan has also presented problems because of the inevitable changes in technique associated with the improvements in scanning equipment during the course of the studies. One must also decide whether reduced activity on a scan represents healing, or merely a reduction in bone turnover– a point which is of particular importance when the response to cytotoxic agents is considered. The relevance or otherwise of changes in acid phosphatase is another factor which requires further study, especially as the conclusions of Paulson et al. (1979) are at variance with those of Merrin et al. (1976), whilst Khan et al. (1977) have noted that changes, at least in bone marrow acid phosphatase, are not necessarily associated with cancer of the prostate.

The importance of this subject has led to the formation of a sub-committee to consider the matter, consisting of members of the EORTC, the British Prostate Study Group, and Dr. Byar of the National Cancer Institute, under the chairmanship of Mr. M.R.G. Robinson of Pontefract. Its formal report is expected to be available for the next meeting of the EORTC Group in June 1980. As part of the process the EORTC Data Center is preparing an analysis of response for patients entered into protocols 30761 and 30762 by T category, M category, and by the use of the ancillary factor-scoring system recommended by Kvols et al. (1977).

7 Chemotherapy in Prostatic Cancer

Since hormonal therapy is not uniformly effective it is of interest to investigate the value of cytotoxic agents in patients who have failed on hormonal treatment, and also perhaps in those patients with poorly differentiated lesions involving a poor prognosis. This approach has gained impetus from the observation of Kliman et al. (1978) that a decreased uptake of ^{3}H-dihydrotestosterone is observed in nodal metastases, suggesting that there are two populations of cells, one hormone-sensitive and one resistant to such therapy.

7.1 National Prostatic Cancer Project

In its clinical studies, the NPCP has concentrated on the evaluation of cytotoxic agents in prostatic cancer, including those compounds combining hormones and cytotoxic drugs (Estracyt and Prednimustine). Ten protocols have now been implemented and are summarised in Table 11. Full details of these studies are available in the paper by Beckley et al. (to be published).

The results of the first four studies (protocols 100–400) have now been reported (Scott et al. 1975; Murphy et al. 1977, 1979; Schmidt et al. 1979). In these studies patients had failed on standard hormonal therapy and were showing evidence of progressive disease. Response has been considered to include all patients showing complete or partial regression *and* those whose disease remained stable whilst on treatment.

In each study a high proportion of patients receiving the cytotoxic agents noted subjective improvement. In the *first study* relief of pain occurred in 54%–64%, and weight gain, increase in haemoglobin, and improvement in performance status in 13%–34% of patients. In the *second study* analysis was based upon the combination of performance status, pain relief, serum acid phosphatase, and tumour reduction. Here the average improvement in the patients receiving chemotherapy was approximately double that seen in those receiving standard therapy, similar to the findings in the first study. In the *third study* subjective assessment was made of pain relief, weight gain, and performance status, but in this study 'responders' included all patients whose performance status had not deteriorated. Patients receiving procarbazine fared significantly worse than those receiving other treatments. In the *fourth study* pain relief and stable or improved performance status were similar in both treatment arms, being seen in approximately one-third of patients.

From these studies there can be little doubt that the use of cytotoxic agents offers considerable potential for the relief of symptoms in these patients.

The assessment of objective response is more controversial, however, since the true remission rate in all these studies is very low and is illustrated by the figures shown in Table 11 for the response rates in protocols 100–400. The question at issue is whether the achievement of stable disease in a patient whose disease was previously considered to be progressing can legitimately be regarded as a response. In favour of such a view is the fact that resolution of bony metastases in patients with prostatic cancer occurs very

Table 11. Analysis of results of NPCP protocols 100–400, with special reference to 'objective response' and the differences between objective response and partial remission

Protocol	Response	Treatment (% results)		
100		Standard	5-Fluorouracil	Cyclophosphamide
	Objective response	19	36	46
	Partial remission	0	12	7
200		Standard	Estracyt	Streptozotocin
	Objective response	16	30	29
	Partial remission	0	5	0
300		Procarbazine	DTIC	Cyclophosphamide
	Objective response	13	24	26
	Partial remission	0	4	0
400		Prednimustine	Prednimustine + Estracyt	
	Objective response	13	13	
	Partial remission	0	2	

slowly even after treatment for limited metastatic disease in relatively fit patients. Patients entered into these studies all had very advanced disease and were in poor general health. In addition, those showing stable disease experienced longer survival than those in whom disease continued to progress. Against it is the fact that progression of bony metastases is also often slow and an assessment of stable disease over a period of weeks or even months would therefore not be unexpected. The validity or otherwise of these observations will become clear as the results of protocols 500, 600, 900, and 1000 emerge. The first evaluation of protocol 500 (Beckley et al. 1979) does, however, suggest that the objective remission rate obtained with DES is probably in the region of 20%.

7.2 Other Chemotherapy Studies

Several other studies have been carried out by different co-operative groups and by individual clinicians, almost all within the last 5 years. The EORTC Urological Group has completed one phase II study comparing adriamycin and procarbazine, and is recruiting patients for a study to assess vindesine.

In EORTC protocol 30763 (Study Co-ordinator J. H. Mulder, Rotterdam), adriamycin 60 mg/m^2 every 3 weeks was compared with procarbazine 200 mg/m^2 on days 1–14 of each 28-day cycle in patients with progressive disease following failure of hormonal therapy. In this study patients were evaluated after two cycles of treatment, at 6–8 weeks. Treatment continued beyond this stage only if objective response was seen. The responses are shown in Table 12 and it will be seen that although the disease remained stable in seven patients only one partial remission occurred. With hindsight it is clear that it would have been preferable to have continued therapy until progression occurred. During the course of this study, however, the gastro-intestinal toxicity of procarbazine was such in the 14 patients treated that entry to this treatment arm was stopped. The final analysis of this study is awaited.

In EORTC Protocol no. 30799 (Co-ordinator Dr. W. Jones, Leeds) patients who have failed on hormone therapy and with marker lesions are being evaluated for response to vindesine, 3.0 mg/m^2 weekly increasing by 0.5 mg/m^2 weekly (subject to toxicity) to a maximum of 4 mg/m^2 weekly. Seven patients have been entered to date.

Table 12. EORTC protocol 30763: Preliminary analysis of response

Response	Adriamycin (25 patients)	Procarbazine (14 patients)
Too early to assess	8	–
Complete remission	–	–
Partial remission	–	1
No change	7	–
Progression	6	5
Early death	4	8
Total	25	14

Since Carter and Wasserman's paper (1975), in which the early work on cytotoxic chemotherapy was assessed, several other studies of single agents and combination regimes have been published. These are summarised in Tables 13 and 14. It seems logical to assume that the results will improve with prolonged therapy in patients at an earlier stage of the disease, but the extent of such benefit is still unclear.
It is imperative to determine, with the information now becoming available from hormonal studies, the minimum duration of cytotoxic chemotherapy required before maximum response rates to the various drugs available are observed. It may be that in patients with advanced and progressive cancer who have already failed on hormone therapy the tumour load may be so great that it is unreasonable to expect objective remissions. Symptomatic relief is seen in many patients, however, and the NPCP studies show a related increase in survival. An immediate objective therefore may be to determine the relationship between relief of symptoms and the length of survival for each cytotoxic agent. It could also be advantageous to evaluate the relative merits of ancillary scoring systems compared with individual factors (e.g., changes in the phosphatases, weight and haemoglobin) in predicting the efficacy of anticancer drugs. Relief of symptoms, delay of progression, and increase in survival are probably the most desirable aims capable of achievement at present.

Table 13. Objective remissions observed with different cytotoxic agents used alone in varying doses

Drug	Remissions evaluable patients	
Adriamycin	21/92 (23%)	Carter and Wasserman (1975); Corder and Cicmil (1976); De Wis (1975); De Wis et al. (1977); Eagan et al. (1976)
cis-Platinum	24/100 (24%)	Merrin (1979); Rossof et al. (1979); Yagoda (1979)
Cyclophosphamide	11/145 (7.6%)	Beckley et al. (1979); Carter and Wasserman (1975)
DTIC	2/61 (3%)	Beckley et al. (1979); Carter and Wasserman (1975)
5-Fluorouracil	23/99 (23%)	Carter and Wasserman (1975); Johnson et al. (1977)
Hydroxyurea	9/38 (24%)	Beckley et al. (1979); Kvols et al. (1977); Lerner et al. (1975)
Methyl-CCNU	1/33 (3%)	Beckley et al. (1979); Carter and Wasserman (1975)
Melphalan	0/35 (0%)	Franks (1979); Houghton et al. (1977); Kvols et al. (1977)
Procarbazine	0/39 (0%)	Beckley et al. (1979)
Vincristine	2/36 (6%)	Beckley et al. (1979); Carter and Wasserman (1975)

Table 14. Responses observed with combinations of cytotoxic agents in patients with prostatic cancer

Combination	Response: Remissions evaluable patients	Stable disease	Subjective response	Survival in responders/ non-responders (days)
Adriamycin + cyclophosphamide				
Merrin et al. (1976)	0/21	5/21	8/21	–
Lloyd et al. (1976)	2/11	–	–	–
Izbicki et al. (1979)	3/20 (10%)	5/20	8/20	280/119
5-Fluorouracil + cyclophosphamide				
Merrin et al. (1976)	1/13	1/13	7/13	–
Eagan et al. (1976)	2/12 (12%)	–	–	273/143
Adriamycin + 5-fluorouracil + cyclophosphamide				
Chlebowski et al. (1978)	0/12	6/12	–	245/303
Soloway et al. (1979)	0/21 (0%)	12/21	5/21	460/204
5-Fluorouracil + methotrexate + vincristine + L-PAM + prednisone				
Kane et al. (1977)	6/25 (24%)	12/25	24/25	441/280

8 Conclusions

1. DES is still the standard hormonal therapy and is effective in relieving symptoms for a time in the majority of patients. The true remission rate is probably in the region of 20%.
2. In the VACURG studies, (a) DES slowed the rate of progression from non-metastatic to metastatic disease, but did not increase survival; (b) orchidectomy and the combination of orchidectomy and DES were not superior to DES alone. It is not yet known whether orchidectomy is superior to DES 1 mg/day in those with or without cardiovascular hazard; (c) undue cardiovascular hazard has not so far been demonstrated in patients with metastatic disease treated with DES; (d) DES 1 mg/day is as effective as DES 5 mg/day in controlling symptoms, and is free from cardiovascular hazard.
3. The current EORTC studies are expected to reveal (a) the cardiovascular hazard of DES 1 mg t.d.s.; and (b) the remission rate with DES 1 mg t.d.s., Estracyt, cyproterone, and Provera.
4. There is as yet little evidence in favour of any form of active treatment for patients presenting with category T0 or T1 disease in the absence of metastases (M0).
5. The evaluation of objective remission in patients with prostatic cancer is difficult and confused. Time to progression and overall survival are easier to determine and probably of greater significance.
6. There is some evidence that the cells of metastases may be less hormone-sensitive than those of the primary tumor, raising the possibility of two cell populations requiring separate forms of therapy.
7. Despite intensive study of cytotoxic chemotherapy in the last 5 years, little clear information has emerged. Further detailed evaluation of criteria of remission is urgently required.
8. It will be possible to evaluate the role of cytotoxic agents more effectively when the results of NPCP protocols 500, 600, 900, and 1,000 are available. Cytotoxic agents can, however, relieve symptoms and prolong survival.

9 References

Beckley S, Wajsman Z, Slack N, Mittelman A, Murphy GP (to be published) The chemotherapy of prostatic carcinoma. Scand J Urol Nephrol

Blackard CE, Mellinger GT, Gleason DF (1971) Treatment of stage 1 carcinoma of the prostate. A preliminary report. J Urol 106: 729–733

Byar DP (1973) The Veterans Administration Cooperative Urological Research Group's studies of cancer of the prostate. Cancer 32: 1126–1130

Byar DP (1980) Review of the Veterans Administration studies of cancer of the prostate and new results concerning treatment of stage I and II tumours. In: Pavone-Macaluso M, Smith PH, Edsmyr F (eds) Bladder tumours and other topics in urological oncology. Plenum Press, New York London, pp 471–492

Byar DP, Veterans Administration Cooperative Urological Research Group (1972) Survival of patients with incidentally found microscopic cancer of the prostate: results of a clinical trial of conservative treatment. J Urol 108: 908–913

Carter SK, Wasserman TH (1975) The chemotherapy of urologic cancer. Cancer 36: 729–747

Chlebowski RT, Hestorff R, Sardoff L, Weiner J, Bateman JR (1978) Cyclophosphamide (NSC 26271) versus the combination of adriamycin (NSC 123127), 5-fluorouracil (NSC 19893), and cylophosphamide in the treatment of metastatic prostatic cancer. A randomised trial. Cancer 42: 2546–2552
Corder MP, Cicmil GA (1976) Effective treatment of metastatic squamous carcinoma of the prostate with adriamycin. J Urol 115: 222
Correa RJ Jr, Anderson RG, Gibbons RP, Mason JT (1974) Latent carcinoma of the prostate – why the controversy? J Urol 111: 644–646
De Wys WD (1975) Comparison of adriamycin (NSC 123127) and 5-fluorouracil (NSC-19893) in advanced prostatic cancer. Cancer Chemother Rep 59: 215–217
De Wys WD, Bauer M, Colsky J, Cooper RA, Creech R, Carbone PP (1977) Comparative trial of adriamycin and 5-fluorouracil in advanced prostatic cancer. Progress report. Cancer Treat Rep 61: 325–328
Donohue RE, Fauver HE, Whitesel JA, Pfister RR (1979) Staging prostatic cancer: a different distribution. J Urol 122: 327–329
Eagan RT, Hahn RG, Myers RP (1976) Adriamycin versus 5FU and cyclophosphamide in the treatment of metastatic prostatic cancer. Cancer Treat Rep 60: 115–117
Franks CR (1979) Melphalan in metastatic cancer of the prostate. Cancer Treat Rev [Suppl] 6: 121–125
Houghton AL, Robinson MRG, Smith PH (1977) Melphalan in advanced prostatic cancer. A pilot study. Cancer Chemother Rep 61: 923–924
Huggins C, Hodges CV (1941) Studies on prostatic cancer. 1. The effect of castration, of estrogen and of androgen injection on serum phosphatases in metastatic carcinoma of the prostate. Cancer Res 1: 293–297
Izbicki RM, Amer MH, Al-Sarraf M (1979) Combination of adriamycin and cyclophosphamide in the treatment of metastatic prostatic carcinoma: A phase II study. Cancer Treat Rep 63: 999–1001
Johnson DE, Scott WW, Gibbons RP, Prout GR Jr, Schmidt JD, Chu TM, Gaeta J, Saroff J, Murphy GP (1977) National randomised study of chemotherapeutic agents in advanced prostatic cancer. A progress report. Cancer Treat Rep 61: 317–323
Jordan WP Jr, Blackard CE, Byar DP (1977) Reconsideration of orchiectomy in the treatment of advanced prostatic carcinoma. South Med J 70: 1411–1413
Kane RD, Stocks LH, Paulson DF (1977) Multiple drug chemotherapy regimen for patients with hormonally-unresponsive carcinoma of the prostate: A preliminary report. J Urol 117: 467–471
Khan R, Turner B, Edson M, Dolan M (1977) Bone marrow acid phosphatase: Another look. J Urol 117: 79–80
Kliman B, Prout GR Jr, Maclaughlin RA, Daly JJ, Griffin PP (1978) Altered androgen metabolism in metastatic prostate cancer. J Urol 119: 623–626
Kvols LK, Eagan RT, Myers RP (1977) Evaluation of melphalan, ICRF-159 and hydroxyurea in metastatic prostatic cancer: A preliminary report. Cancer Treat Rep 61: 311–312
Lerner H, Malloy T, Cromie W, Longo S (1975) Hydroxyurea in stage D carcinoma of the prostate. A pilot study. J Urol 114: 425–429
Lloyd RE, Jones SE, Salmon SE, Durie BGM, McMahon LJ (1976) Combination chemotherapy with adriamycin (NSC-123127) and cyclophosphamide (NSC-26271) for solid tumors: A phase II trial. Cancer Treat Rep 60: 77–83
Menon M, Walsh PC (1979) Hormonal therapy for prostatic cancer. In: Murphy GP (ed) Prostatic cancer. P.S.G., Littleton, pp 175–200
Merrin CE (1979) Treatment of genitourinary tumors with *cis*-dichlorodiammineplatinum. II. Experience in 250 patients. Cancer Treat Rep 63: 1579–1584
Merrin C, Etra W, Wajsman Z, Baumgartner G, Murphy G (1976) Chemotherapy of advanced carcinoma of the prostate with 5-fluorouracil, cyclophosphamide and adriamycin. J Urol 115: 86–88

Murphy GP, Gibbons RP, Johnson DE, Loening SA, Prout GR, Schmidt JD, Bross DS, Chu TM, Gaeta JF, Saroff J, Scott, WW (1977) A Comparison of estramustine phosphate and streptozotocin in patients with advanced prostatic carcinoma who have had extensive irradiation. J Urol 118: 288–291

Murphy GP, Gibbons RP, Johnson DE, Prout GR, Schmidt JD, Soloway MS, Loening SA, Chu TM, Gaeta JF, Saroff J, Wajsman Z, Slack N, Scott WW (1979) The use of estramustine and prednimustine versus prednimustine alone in advanced metastatic prostatic cancer patients who have received prior irradiation. J Urol 121: 763–765

Paulson DF, Berry WR, Cox EB, Walker A, Laszlo J (1979) Treatment of metastatic endocrine-unresponsive carcinoma of the prostate gland with multiagent chemotherapy: Indicators of response to therapy. J Natl Cancer Inst 63: 615–622

Robinson MRG, Thomas BG (1971) Effect of hormonal therapy on plasma testosterone levels in prostatic carcinoma. Br Med J 4: 391–394

Rossof AH, Talley RW, Stephens R, Thigpen T, Samson MK, Groppe C Jr, Eyre, HJ, Fisher R (1979) Phase II evaluation of *cis*-dichlorodiammineplatinum (II) in advanced malignancies of the genitourinary and gynecologic organs: A Southwest Oncology Group study. Cancer Treat Rep 63: 1557–1564

Schmidt JD, Scott WW, Gibbons RP, Johnson DE, Prout GR Jr, Loening SA, Soloway MS, Chu TM, Gaeta JF, Slack NH, Saroff J, Murphy GP (1979) Comparison of procarbazine, imidazole-carboxamide and cyclophosphamide in relapsing patients with advanced carcinoma of the prostate. J Urol 121: 185–189

Scott WW, Johnson DE, Schmidt JE, Gibbons RP, Prout GR, Joiner JR, Saroff J, Murphy GP (1975) Chemotherapy of advanced prostatic carcinoma with cyclophosphamide or 5-fluorouracil: Results of the First National Randomized Study. J Urol 114: 909–911

Silverberg GD (1977) Hypophysectomy in the Treatment of Disseminated Prostate Carcinoma. Cancer 39: 1727–1731

Smith PH (to be published) The medical management of prostatic cancer – some current questions. Eur Urol

Soloway MS, Shippel RM, Ikard M (1979) Cyclophosphamide, doxorubicin hydrochloride and 5-fluorouracil in advanced carcinoma of the prostate. J Urol 122: 637–639

Veterans Administration Cooperative Urological Research Group (1967) Treatment and survival of patients with cancer of the prostate. Surg Gynecol Obstet 124: 1011–1017

Wynder El, Mabuchi K, Whitmore WF Jr (1971) Epidemiology of cancer of the prostate. Cancer 28: 344–360

Yagoda A (1979) Phase II trials with *cis*-dichlorodiammineplatinum (II) in the treatment of urothelial cancer. Cancer Treat Rep 63: 1565–1572

Perspectives and Prospects

G. D. Chisholm

Department of Surgery (Urology), University of Edinburgh, GB – Edinburgh

1 Introduction

To give a tumour perspective is to consider both its impact on society and its impact on the patient. The estimated incidence of carcinoma of the prostate in the United Kingdom is 5,700 new cases per year (Tate et al. 1979); it is the sixth most common malignancy overall, but the commonest cancer of the male genito-urinary tract. In the United States there are 42,000 new cases per year and this tumour is the second most common cause of cancer deaths (Klein 1979). Despite such an incidence, carcinoma of the prostate is a malignancy which lacks popular image. Just as benign prostatic hyperplasia is often relegated to 'only an old man's problem', so it is that the malignant prostate has little impact on general discussions on cancer. Indeed a number of tumours with a lower incidence have more appeal and, therefore, have larger resources devoted to them.

2 Perspectives

It will be acknowledged that because of improved life expectancy there is an increasing older population more likely to be affected by carcinoma of the prostate. Thus in Scotland in 1930–1932, life expectancy for a male at birth was 56 years, whereas by 1970–1972 life expectancy at birth had increased to 67.2 years. There is now some evidence that the increase in the proportion of elderly persons in the population may have reached a plateau and the projected population changes in Scotland over the next 10 years are shown in Table 1. However, since the over 65-year-olds account for approximately one-eighth of the total male population in Scotland, there are good

Table 1. Projected population in Scotland for males over 65. Lothian Health Board Report (1978)

1977	267,300
1981	275,300
1986	273,700
1991	278,000

Recent Results in Cancer Research, Vol. 78
© Springer-Verlag Berlin · Heidelberg 1981

reasons for ensuring that, despite their age, these men receive the optimum treatment for carcinoma of the prostate.

Considerable debate has been engendered over the apparent lack of progress in diagnosing and treating some malignancies. For example, it is suggested that despite all efforts, the mortality and morbidity for many malignant tumours have not changed over the past 50 years. While this may be true for some tumours such as carcinoma of the breast, this suggestion must be put in perspective. Indeed it may not now be true for carcinoma of the breast (Haybittle 1979), and it certainly does not apply to a great many other tumours, such as the testicular tumours (Johnson et al. 1980). An answer to any of these challenges requires reliable data and it is these or the lack of these data, that weaken so many discussions.

2.1 Improvement in Survival Rates

Recently the statistics concerning carcinoma of the prostate have been examined by Enstrom and Austin (1977). These authors point out that in the United States there was no organised system for collection of data on cancer until 1956. Hence the End Results Evaluation Program (EREP) began in 1956 (Cutler and Latourette 1959) and the California Tumor Registry (CTR) was established in 1947. In their study of cancer survival rates Enstrom and Austin have shown that there have been substantial improvements in survival for carcinoma of the prostate. Table 2 shows their comparison of the incidence and mortality rates for white males in 1950 and 1970. These data show an improvement in the 5-year survival rate from 30%–59%, i.e., the rate has almost doubled in 20 years. The explanation for this change is a sharp increase in the number of new patients that have either occult or early tumours, which are also those that should have a better prognosis. It is possible that an increase in the number of autopsies and earlier operations for outflow tract obstructive symptoms have also led to an increase in the recorded incidence (Klein 1979).

Thus the increase in the survival rate for patients with carcinoma of the prostate has occurred because the *incidence rate* has increased markedly while the *mortality rate* has shown a negligible decline, and this has led Enstrom and Austin (1977) to conclude that we need a better guide to progress in the management of a tumour (or disease) than survival rates and that a more helpful expression of this progress needs to be derived from incidence and mortality rates.

2.2 Importance of Early Diagnosis

In consideration of these data we can also recognise a painful truism, that in order to see a disease in perspective we are wholly dependent on good records and good disease

Table 2. Five-year survival rates for carcinoma of the prostate 1950 and 1970. Klein (1979)

	1950	1970
Incidence per million	17	21
Mortality per million (age adjusted)	7.5	7.0
5-Year survival rate	30%	59%

classifications. Only in more recent years has any serious attempt been made to collect such data.

Several questions arise from the foregoing comments:

1. *What is the extent of the suggested increase in early/occult carcinoma of the prostate?* A decade or more ago the majority of reports on the incidence of stage A or 1 disease showed figures that ranged from 5%–16% (Varkarakis et al. 1970). Data from the California Tumor Registry now show that over a period of about 30 years there has been a 50% increase in the diagnosis of localised prostatic cancer (Table 3). Other recent reports have also shown an increase in the proportion of early-stage carcinoma of the prostate at the time of diagnosis (McMillen and Wettlaufer 1976; Donohue et al. 1979). In a review of 100 consecutive new patients in the Department of Surgery, University of Edinburgh, there were 23% T0 cases, and only 1% T1, the remaining T2, T3, and T4 cases accounting for 76% (Table 4).
2. *Is there an explanation for this increase in the proportion of early-stage tumours?* In our society it is very uncommon for a well man to undergo a physical examination that includes a rectal examination. Experience from North America suggests that this form of screening can increase the detection rate of early cancer, but obviously not the occult form; it also seems unlikely that this could be the explanation for the increasing incidence in the negro population in the United States. Self-examination has been suggested from time to time (Lehrer 1978) but has not gained much support. However, an awareness of altered urinary habits and a willingness to seek advice could be relevant in bringing forward those patients who are found to have early-stage carcinoma of the prostate. This view is supported in respect of the presentation of the 100 patients already noted in the Edinburgh series. Table 5 shows that nine of ten patients in this series presented with either symptoms of prostatism or retention of urine.
   It seems likely that good urological services, relatively short waiting lists, and a willingness to treat patients with prostatic symptoms early by transurethral resection are also important contributory factors in the diagnosis of early stage tumours.
3. *If patients are presenting at an earlier stage/category, then these patients are those with a better prognosis; do mortality rates reflect this change?* It is not yet possible to give data to support this statement, since the increased incidence rate is a relatively

Table 3. Presentation of carcinoma of the prostate in patients from the California Tumor Registry. Klein (1979)

Category	Localised	Regional	Distant	Unknown
1942–1954	41	16	28	15
1955–1969	63	13	19	5

Table 4. Carcinoma of the prostate: T category at presentation in 100 new patients

Category	T0	T1	T2	T3	T4
No. of patients	23	1	13	52	11

Table 5. Carcinoma of the prostate: presenting features in 100 new patients

	%
Prostatism	70
Urinary retention	23
Back pain	14
Haematuria	5
Post-prostatectomy symptoms	5
Renal failure	4
Weight loss	3
Altered bowel habit	3
Anaemia	1
Abnormal excretion urogram	1

Table 6. Carcinoma of the prostate: incidence of metastatic disease in early (T0, T1) and locally extensive (T2, T3, T4) disease

T category	No. of patients	M category	
		M0 %	M1 %
T0, T1	24	68	32
T2, T3, T4	76	39	61

Table 7. Carcinoma of the prostate: 5-year corrected survival data for Scotland (1966–1977)

Age (year)	No. of patients	Corrected 5-year survival rate (%)
45–54	19	35.3
55–64	151	43.4
65–74	453	45.6
75–84	395	28.1
Over 85	86	20.7

Table 8. Carcinoma of the prostate: 10-year survival rates with different age groups. Axtell et al. (1972)

Age (years)	10-Year survival rate (%)	
	All patients	Local disease
45–54	37	55
55–64	30	41
65–74	17	22
Over 75	5	6

Table 9. Five-year survival rates for the eight most common cancers. Tate et al. (1979)

Tumour site	5-Year survival rate (%)
Breast	49
Cervix	47
Bladder	35
Colon and rectum	28
Prostate	27
Lung	5
Stomach	5
Pancreas	1

recent trend. However, this evidence should be forthcoming, since it is well established that patients with focal, incidentally diagnosed carcinoma of the prostate have a survival rate similar to that of a matched population and rarely die from their malignancy (Byar 1977).

Although early-stage tumours can have a good prognosis, this group is heterogeneous, and Barnes et al. (1976) have emphasised that a substantial proportion of patients with stage A and B tumours may die from their disease. In the Edinburgh series of 100 consecutive new patients one-third of the "early" cases had evidence of metastatic disease at the time of presentation (Table 6), so that it cannot be assumed that patients with early-stage disease are either a uniform group or have an entirely benign prognosis.

4. *Does presentation at an earlier stage/category imply that these are also younger patients?* Again this has not been the author's experience: several studies in the past decade have had a mean age of about 70 years and in the current series under study in Edinburgh the mean age of T0 and T1 cases was 69 years and that for T2, T3, and T4 cases was 71 years.
5. *Is age alone relevant to a discussion on survival?* There is a clinical impression that younger patients often have a worse prognosis. While this may be so for an individual, and especially for a poor-grade tumour, published data have revealed that the overall prognosis for younger patients tends to be better (Tables 7 and 8).
6. *Is carcinoma of the prostate a relatively mild form of cancer?* If 5-year survival data are used to give some perspective to the impact of this tumour on a patient, we see that carcinoma of the prostate has the fifth-best 5-year survival rate of the eight most common cancers (Table 9).

2.3 Assessment of Morbidity

Morbidity is more difficult to quantify, especially in an age group of the population that is already prone to a variety of medical problems. Apart from the difficulties with micturition (Table 5), carcinoma of the prostate characteristically causes bone metastases and these can be extremely painful. The side-effects of oestrogen treatment, which include depression and gynaecomastia, are generally under-rated, and the reaction to the proposal of an orchidectomy can range from stoical acceptance to outright refusal to have such an operation.

It is true that these patients are not usually affected in the so-called prime of life, as for example patients with testicular tumours are, but then carcinoma of the prostate is some 15 times more common than testicular tumours, and many men in their fifties to sixties could well argue that *they* are still in their prime of life. Thus a patient with carcinoma of the prostate can have a quality of life that ranges from completely normal to one of severe handicap due to urinary difficulties, including incontinence, bone pain, and cachexia.

3 Prospects

In considering the prospects for carcinoma of the prostate, we shall look at the future in terms of the main subject headings of epidemiology, diagnosis, pathology, and treatment. The next decade will undoubtedly be notable for the limits on money available for both medical care and research. These limits tend to affect first those aspects of medical care that are easily quantifiable. Thus, capital expenditure on new equipment for investigation will be restricted and, to name an obvious example, the CT scanner will remain limited to only a small number of centres in the United Kingdom. Drug costs are equally easy to determine, so that the use of very expensive drugs can only be justified if there are proven clinical advantages. Again, to cite the more obvious, many of the chemotherapy drugs will need to have proven advantages based on comparative clinical trials before their widespread use can be justified. In times of financial restriction, money for medical research is all too readily a target for economy. This past decade has seen a substantial increase in the number of research projects and persons studying the prostate gland. Topics include androgen metabolism (Morfin et al. 1979), binding or 'receptor' proteins of the prostate (Sirett and Grant 1978), experimental models for prostate growth (de Klerk et al. 1979), and prostate organ culture (Lasnitski 1976). Much of the impetus for these projects has come from the availability of radio-immunoassay methods for measuring the steroids involved in the control and growth of the prostate. The clinical relevance of this type of work is gradually emerging, and only with continued support for this type of research can we expect to establish more rational and more effective treatment for this tumour.

3.1 Epidemiology

Since 1941, when Huggins and Hodges concluded that malignancy represented an overgrowth of adult prostatic epithelium, the relationship between benign hyperplasia and malignancy has been debated. There have been two conflicting epidemiological studies, one showing a substantially increased risk of carcinoma in a patient with benign prostatic hyperplasia (Armenian et al. 1974), the other showing no association between the two conditions (Greenwald et al. 1974). The fact that there is an increasing incidence of occult focal cancer with age in the benign prostate continues to support the view that there may be factors common to both benign and malignant change. However, the striking differences in the prostatic cancer death rates between, for example, Japanese and United States blacks suggest that factors other than or in addition to age affect the prostate. From a comparison of blacks in Washington, DC and in West Africa, it appears that external environmental factors other than racial origin affect the development of carcinoma in the prostate (Jackson et al. 1977). Even within the United States, blacks have an extremely high incidence rate compared with other racial-ethnic groups.

With such striking epidemiological differences there must now be a real prospect of identifying the risk factors affecting the prostate and of resolving the debate over the hypotheses concerning the aetiology of carcinoma of the prostate (Ross et al. 1979).

3.2 Diagnosis

Approximately 60% of patients with carcinoma of the prostate have locally advanced tumours, and 50% of all patients presenting with carcinoma of the prostate have evidence of metastatic disease at the time of presentation. The prospect of reducing this high proportion of advanced disease must be the aim for the next decade. The majority of patients seek medical advice only because of symptoms of prostatism. It has been suggested that a shorter history of prostatism is more likely to indicate malignancy but this is not a reliable observation and offers little prospect of practical use in obtaining an earlier diagnosis. Similarly, well-man screening seems unlikely to be extended in the United Kingdom beyond some insurance examinations and the few private clinics which offer this service. Even if a regular rectal examination of the prostate were to be carried out, the examining finger will not detect focal carcinoma, and as Jewett (1975) has pointed out, there is a significant error rate in diagnosis of malignant nodules by rectal examination alone.

Despite the limitations in the use of serum acid phosphatase in the diagnosis of metastatic carcinoma of the prostate, this enzyme remains the best available marker for this tumour. The prospect of improving its sensitivity by radio-immunoassay, counter-immune electrophoresis, or immunofluoroassay can be confidently expected from the preliminary data already published (Wajsman et al. 1979). The role of these more sensitive methods in screening apparently normal patients offers the further prospect of detecting early asymptomatic disease.

The confirmation of diagnosis by biopsy is unlikely to be superseded by the Franzén needle aspiration method: the cytological expertise required for the latter is not widely available throughout the United Kingdom. Techniques for studying the aspirated cells by cytophotometric DNA analysis (Zetterberg and Esposti 1976) or by computerised nuclear morphometry (Stenkvist et al. 1978) offer the prospect of objective measurement of the tumour cells, which may then be correlated with tumour progression and prognosis.

Interest continues to grow in the use of the improved imaging techniques that are now available. Transabdominal and perineal ultrasound are not sufficiently sensitive but transurethral and transrectal real-time scans are proving more precise. Peeling et al. (1979) have already shown how the rectal probe can be used to give a reliable indication of any capsular invasion, especially of the anteriorly placed tumours. Computed tomography has, so far, proved disappointing in defining the margins of the prostate (this volume, Chap. 6).

3.3 Pathology

The pathologist will continue to be the key person in providing basic information on the tumour from which treatment decisions can then be made. If we know the precise staging of the tumour and its grade, management can be rationalised. However, we must be aware of the constraints that examination of the prostate places on the pathologist. In particular, how many sections of the tissue received must be studied before giving an opinion? This problem has become accentuated by the difficulty in diagnosing focal carcinoma from a prostatectomy specimen removed by transurethral resection.

The classification of focal carcinoma in the TNM system is not satisfactory; the difference between a few foci of carcinoma cells and diffuse involvement is not clear from the T or pT category. The Whitmore (1956) system, according to which incidentally diagnosed carcinoma of the prostate is stage A, has now been extended, so that $A1_F$ is focal carcinoma, A1 is limited to one lobe, and A2 denotes diffuse involvement. It is in this group of focal tumours that we look for clarification in the future. Should a second resection be mandatory to determine the extent of invasion? Should we be looking for other methods for determining the extent of tumour in the resected tissue? The prospect for sorting out the stage/category of the tumour will require a very close liaison between urologist and pathologist to reach a conclusion. The reason why such a refinement of classification is necessary must be emphasised. It is because the prognosis for some focal carcinomas is so good that many urologists would prefer to defer treatment – provided that the tumour really is focal. The prospect for the 1980s is to see this problem resolved, and hopefully there will emerge a combination of the focal category and the tumour grade that will give a clearer indication of the biological potential of the tumour.

It may be that characterisation of receptor proteins will be necessary to provide this answer (this volume, Chap. 4). However, the technological problems in studying small samples of prostatic tissue seem to be of such magnitude that alternative techniques must be developed to characterise these tissues.

3.4 Treatment

The prospect for treatment in the future is an end to the doubts about the correct choice of treatment for each of the different stages/grades of the disease.

3.4.1 Localised Disease

Comment has been made already on the problems relating to the diagnosis of focal carcinoma. The management of this stage of the disease has created such doubt that the Medical Research Council has encouraged a clinical trial of T0/T1 NXM0 tumours to resolve the question of whether early cancer of the prostate should be treated with radiotherapy or whether a policy of deferred treatment of the primary tumour is safe. This trial will compare immediate radical radiotherapy only (either 5,000 rads in 20 fractions in 4 weeks, or 6,000 rads in 30 fractions in 6 weeks) with deferred treatment, that is no active treatment will be given until progression of the tumour is evident.

The prospect of rationalising the management of more advanced but still localised prostatic cancer (T2, T3 or T4, NXM0) will depend on the outcome of the second Medical Research Council trial for prostatic cancer. This trial aims to resolve whether orchidectomy, radical radiotherapy, or a combination of these treatments delays the appearance of metastases and prolongs survival.

Table 10. Comparison of survival rates with different forms of treatment for carcinoma of the prostate. Chisholm (1980)

Treatment	Stage	Survival (years)		
		5	10	15
Radical prostatectomy (Jewett 1975)	B1			33
	B2			18
Endocrine treatment (Barnes and Ninan 1972)	A + B		57	33
Radical prostatectomy (Schröder and Belt 1975)	C		36	20
Radiotherapy (Bagshaw et al. 1977)	B	70	42	
	C	36	29	
Radiotherapy (Harisiadis et al. 1978)	A	88		
	B	87		
	C	58		
	Overall	40	64	

Table 11. Carcinoma of the prostate: 5-year survival rates following interstitial ^{125}I as primary treatment. W. F. Whitmore (1979, personal communication)

Stage[a]	5-year survival rate
B (N−)	100%
B (N+)	90%
C (N−)	90% (30% with M+)
C (N+)	70% (50% with M+)

[a] N, pelvic lymph nodes; M, distant metastases

It will be seen from both these trials that radiotherapy has now gained an important place in the primary management of carcinoma of the prostate. The results from centres with long-term experience with this treatment show results that match any of the other forms of treatment for this tumour (Table 10).

The question that will need to be resolved is whether or not interstitial iodine-125 has significant advantages over supervoltage radiotherapy. So far, the experience with over 400 patients at the Memorial Hospital, New York, has shown very good results (Table 11). Because of these results, it is already evident that a clinical trial to compare interstitial with external beam therapy is unlikely. The challenge is, therefore, for other centres to achieve better results with new techniques based on particulate radiations such as protons, pions, or fast neutrons.

3.4.2 Generalised Disease

The primary care for a patient who presents with metastatic disease is the use of some form of endocrine manipulation (Chisholm 1980). Stilboestrol easily holds its position as the most cost-effective drug; the precise dose has yet to be resolved. A dose of 1 mg per day may be enough, but 1 mg t.d.s. suppresses serum testosterone more uniformly and for this reason this dose has gained popular acceptance. Whether this difference in dose affects survival rates is not known, nor do we know the cardiovascular complication rate associated with these two dose levels.

A more pressing question to resolve is whether or not orchidectomy is the endocrine treatment of choice, or whether the combination of stilboestrol plus orchidectomy might be the best approach (de Vere White et al. 1977). One can only express surprise that 40 years after Huggins and Hodges (1941) advocated endocrine treatment, there is still uncertainty as to the best form this should take. There is no doubt, however, that the adverse effects of high-dose oestrogens have led to renewed interest in the advantages of an orchidectomy; a subcapsular orchidectomy has been shown to be a complete castration (Clark and Houghton 1977) and this may be preferred by both urologist and patient.

Much effort and money is spent in finding an alternative to stilboestrol. In general these efforts have been disappointing, and current trials by groups such as EORTC and the British Prostate Group may also be disappointing, because each trial requires such large numbers and such a long follow-up to obtain statistically significant results. Nevertheless, the place of any other drug in the primary treatment of carcinoma of the prostate must be established from clinical trials (see this volume, Chap. 11). Tate et al. (1979) have pointed out how few patients with carcinoma of the prostate are entered into any clinical trial in the United Kingdom.

The final prospect is that the treatment of that most difficult group of all, those patients who escape endocrine control, will improve. The objective criteria for recognising that a tumour is no longer sensitive to endocrine treatment are few. The clinician must rely on rectal findings, serum acid phosphatase, and the bone scan. A definition of the various degrees of regression and progression is essential for a patient entered into a clinical trial, but in general these criteria are difficult to apply and unnecessarily complex in practice. The hope is that these criteria can be simplified and made more reliable.

The wide choice of treatment for the 'oestrogen escape' patient indicates the relatively poor response rate to all of them. A small group of cytotoxic drugs has now been shown to be active against carcinoma of the prostate; their role in the care of these patients now needs to be defined. So far, with cytotoxic drugs used as single agents the response rates have been approximately 20% objective and 40% subjective responses. We now face the prospect of combination chemotherapy to improve these results.

Indeed, it may be that the time has now come to consider the planned progression of a combination of these treatments. For example, a patient with a localised tumour (M0) might receive radiotherapy (to the pelvis) and chemotherapy (for micrometastases) and have endocrine therapy reserved for symptomatic metastases. There is now good reason for such a programme of treatment to be seriously considered.

Patients with carcinoma of the prostate are receiving more attention than in the past and, in some urological centres, 'prostate clinics' are held to monitor these patients more carefully and to change treatment when indicated. A 'wait and see' approach to this tumour is no longer acceptable unless under close supervision, and although much of the treatment remains palliative, a better quality of life can now be assured for most of these patients.

4 References

Armenian HK, Lilienfeld AM, Diamond EL, Bross ID (1974) Relation between benign prostatic hyperplasia and cancer of the prostate. A prospective and retrospective study. Lancet 2: 115–117

Axtell LM, Cutler SJ, Myers MH (eds) (1972) End results in cancer. Government Printing Office, Washington (Report no. 4, Department of Health, Education and Welfare; Publication no. (NIH) 73–272, National Cancer Institute)

Bagshaw MA, Pistenma DA, Ray GR (1977) Evaluation of extended-field radiotherapy for prostate neoplasms: 1976 progress report. Cancer Treat Rep 61: 297–306

Barnes RW, Hirst A, Rosenquist R (1976) Early carcinoma of the prostate: comparison of stages A and B. J Urol 115: 404–405

Barnes RW, Ninan CA (1972) Carcinoma of the prostate: biopsy and conservative therapy. J Urol 108: 897–900

Byar DP (1977) VACURG studies on prostatic cancer and its treatment. In: Tannenbaum M (ed) Urologic pathology: the prostate. Lea & Febiger, New York, pp 241–267

Chisholm GD (1980) Malignancy: prostate. In: Chisholm GD (ed) Tutorials in postgraduate medicine: urology. Heinemann, London, pp 223–246

Clark P, Houghton L (1977) Subcapsular orchidectomy for carcinoma of the prostate. Br J Urol 49: 419–425

Cutler SJ, Latourette HB (1959) A national cooperative program for the evaluation of end results in cancer. J Natl Cancer Inst 22: 633–646

de Klerk DP, Coffey DS, Ewing LL, McDermott IR, Reiner WG, Robinson CH, Scott WW, Strandberg JD, Talalay P, Walsh PC, Wheaton LG, Zirkin BR (1979) Comparison of spontaneous and experimentally induced canine prostatic hyperplasia. J Clin Invest 64: 842–849

de Vere White R, Paulson DF, Glenn JF (1977) The clinical spectrum of prostate cancer. J Urol 117: 323–327

Donohue RE, Fauver HE, Whitesel JA, Pfister RR (1979) Staging prostatic cancer: a different distribution. J Urol 122: 327–329

Enstrom JE, Austin DF (1977) Interpreting cancer survival rates. Science 195: 847–851

Greenwald P, Kirmss V, Polan AK, Dick VS (1974) Cancer of the prostate among men with benign prostatic hyperplasia. J Natl Cancer Inst 53: 335–340

Harisiadis L, Veenema RJ, Senyszyn JJ, Puchner PJ, Tretter P, Romas NA, Chang CH, Lattimer JK, Tannenbaum M (1978) Carcinoma of the prostate: treatment with external radiotherapy. Cancer 41: 2131–2142

Haybittle JL (1979) Results of treatment of female breast cancer in the Cambridge area 1960–71. Br J Cancer 40: 56–61

Huggins C, Hodges CV (1941) Studies on prostatic cancer. I. The effect of castration, of estrogen and of androgen injection on serum phosphatases in metastatic carcinoma of the prostate. Cancer Res 1: 293–297

Jackson MA, Ahluwalia BS, Herson J (1977) Characterisation of prostatic carcinoma among blacks: a continuation report. Cancer Treat Rep 61: 167–172

Jewett HJ (1975) The present status of radical prostatectomy for stages A and B prostatic cancer. Urol Clin North Am 2: 105–124

Johnson DE, Hussey DH, Samuels ML (1980) Malignancy: testis. In: Chisholm GD (ed) Tutorials in postgraduate medicine: urology. Heinemann, London, pp 247–265

Klein LA (1979) Prostatic carcinoma. N Engl J Med 300: 824–833

Lasnitski I (1976) Action of hormones on the normal prostate and prostatic tumours grown in vitro. In: Williams DI, Chisholm GD (eds) Scientific foundations of urology. Heinamann, London, pp 365–370

Lehrer S (1978) Rectal self-examination. Am J Dig Dis 23: 572–573

Lothian Health Board (1978) Annual statistical report. Lothian Health Board, Edinburgh

McMillen SM, Wettlaufer JN (1976) The role of repeat transurethral biopsy in Stage A carcinoma of the prostate. J Urol 116: 759–760
Morfin RF, Charles J-F, Floch HH (1979) $C_{19}O_2$-Steroid transformations in the human normal, hyperplastic and cancerous prostate. J Steroid Biochem 11: 599–607
Peeling WB, Griffiths GJ, Evans KT, Roberts EE (1979) Diagnosis and staging of prostatic cancer by transrectal ultrasonography. A preliminary study. Br J Urol 51: 565–569
Ross RK, McCurtis JW, Henderson BE, Menck HR, Mack TM, Martin SP (1979) Descriptive epidemiology of testicular and prostatic cancer in Los Angeles. Br J Cancer 39: 284–292
Schröder FH, Belt E (1975) Carcinoma of the prostate: a study of 213 patients with stage C tumors treated by total perineal prostatectomy. J Urol 114: 257–267
Sirett DAN, Grant JK (1978) Androgen binding in cytosols and nuclei of human benign hyperplastic prostatic tissue. J Endocrinol 77: 101–110
Stenkvist B, Westman-Naeser S, Holmquist J, Nordin B, Bengtsson E, Vegelius J, Eriksson O, Fox CH (1978) Computerized nuclear morphometry as an objective method for characterizing human cancer cell populations. Cancer Res 38: 4688–4697
Tate HC, Rawlinson JB, Freedman LS (1979) Randomised comparative studies in the treatment of cancer in the United Kingdom: room for improvement? Lancet 2: 623–625
Varkarakis M, Castro JE, Azzopardi JG (1970) Prognosis of Stage 1 carcinoma of the prostate. Proc R Soc Med 63: 91–93
Wajsman Z, Chu TM, Saroff J, Slack N, Murphy GP (1979) Two new, direct and specific methods of acid phosphatase determination. Urology 13: 8–11
Whitmore WF Jr (1956) Hormone therapy in prostatic cancer. Am J Med 21: 697–713
Zetterberg A, Esposti P-L (1976) Cytophotometric DNA-analysis of aspirated cells from prostatic carcinoma. Acta Cytol (Baltimore) 20: 46–57

Subject Index

acid phosphatase 11, 14, 55, 115
– counter-immune electrophoresis 179
– immunofluoroassay 179
– in ductal carcinoma 69
– in endometrioid carcinoma 71
– radio-immune assay screening 14
– sensitivity 115
– and staging 125
acinar carcinoma 60, 65
adenocarcinoma 60
– endometrioid 71
– experimental rats 34
– ploidy 32
– – mitotic index 32
– poorly differentiated 32
– – mitotic index 32
– well differentiated 62, 65
adenoid cystic carcinoma 72
adenoma 32, 80
adjuvant management, chemotherapy 149
– irradiation 148
adrenalectomy 129, 160
adriamycin 149, 167, 168, 169
aetiological factors 2f
– –, hormones 44
alcohol 11
alkaline phosphatase 115
aminoglutethimide 129
anatomy 20
– comparative 21
– developmental 20
– normal 20
– human 23
– primate 21
androgen receptors 38
androgens, cell cycle 36
–, – production 38
–, dependence 44
androstenediols 50
androstenedione 45
anti-androgen therapy 44, 160
antibodies, radio-active labelled 109
arteriography 77, 78
aspiration biopsy 32
assay of acid phosphatase, radio-immune 50
– – –, protamine sulphate precipitation 51
– of steroid receptors 50
assessment of response 20
– by bone scanning 115
– by clinical methods 165
– by radiology 92
atrophy 25

beer 11
benign hyperplasia 7, 10, 21, 23
– –, diagnostic radiology 84, 94
– –, hormone stimulation 44
– –, malignant change 23, 178
– –, mitotic rate 35
– –, sonography 84
– –, spermine levels 51
– –, thymidine labelling 35
– –, tissue culture 36
biochemical tumour markers 44
biopsy techniques 32, 67, 121
– –, after radiotherapy 136, 137
– –, Franzén needle 121
– –, Tru-Cut needle 121
bladder cancer 69
bleomycin, scanning agent 108
blood groups 6
bone metastases 108, 110
– site distribution 112
– –, pathological type 77
– –, response to treatment 167
– abnormal scans 112
– accuracy 111
– agents 110
– equipment 110

– mechanisms 110
– scanning 110
breast cancer and prostatic cancer 50
British Prostatic Group 55, 182
Broder's grading 62

cadmium exposure 12
calculi 86
California Tumor registry 174
cancer aetiology 2f
– classification 60f
– latent 2, 45, 157
– generalized 181
– microscopic 45
– origin 25
carcinoembryonic antigen 56
carcinoid tumours 60, 71
carcinoma-in-situ 26
cell cycle, phases 39
– –, time 36
– loss factor 29
– population kinetics 29
– production rate 29
central zone 22
chemotherapy, see cytotoxic chemotherapy
chorionic gonadotrophin 56
cigarette smoking 11
circumcision 9
cis-Platinum 168
clonogenic assay 34
combination chemotherapy 168f
combined management, irradiation and hormones 146
– –, – and orchidectomy 147
– –, – and surgery 148
– –, surgery and hormones 154
comparative anatomy 21
computed tomography 77, 87ff
– techniques 87
– tissue characterisation 88
computerised nuclear morphometry 179
cortisone 129
cyclophosphamide 149, 155, 166, 168, 169
cyproterone acetate 156, 160, 163
cystography 77, 78
cysto-urethrography 77, 78
cytology, diagnosis 121
–, prostatic massage smears 14
–, urine 14
–, transrectal aspiration 14
cytophotometric analysis 179
cytoxan, see cyclophosphamide
cytotoxic chemotherapy 154f
– future role 182
– phased trials 161

dacarbazine 168
dehydroepiandrosterone 45
delay in treatment 145
depostat 160
depression 177
diagnosis, cytological 121
–, digital examination 119
–, early 86, 179
–, histological 60f
–, transurethral resection 120
–, ultrasound 120
diet 10
di-ethyl stilboestrol, see stilboestrol
diffuse carcinoma, management 150, 180
– –, pathology 65
– –, results of treatment 158
dihydrotestosterone 50
–, action on prostate 38
–, cell proliferation 38
–, hormone therapy 160
diphosphonate scanning agents 110
DNA, content in prostatic cancer 33
– synthesis 37
dose radiation 140
– –, tumour control 140
DTIC, see dacarbazine
ductal carcinoma 60
– comedo 70
– cribriform 70
– papillary 70
– primary 69
– secondary 70
duct epithelium 64
– carcinoma 69f
– squamous metaplasia 67

early detection 86, 174
embryology 20
emotional status 11
endocrine ablation 129
– –, testis 147
– –, adrenals 129, 160
– –, pituitary 129, 160
– administration 154f
– –, anti-androgens 44, 160
– –, prednisone 169
– –, progestogens 160, 163f
– –, oestrogens 155, 160f
– –, survival rates 181
endometrioid carcinoma 71

End Results Evaluation Program 174
environmental hazards 13
EORTC Urological Group 163, 167
epidemiology 1, 178
Estracyt 155, 156, 160, 164, 166
ethinyl estradiol 160
ethnic groups 6
– –, Europeans 7
– –, Indians, Americans 7
– –, Japanese 6
– –, Jewish 9
– –, Polish 7
– –, USA 7
excretion urography, see intravenous urography
experimental prostatic tumours 34
external beam radiotherapy, see radiotherapy

flow cytometry 33
5-fluoro-uracil 149, 166, 168, 169
focal carcinoma 120, 158, 180
– –, management 150
– –, pathology 65
Franzén needle 67, 121

gallium bleomycin 108
gamma camera 111
generalised disease, management 159, 181
genetic factors 6
Gleason's grading 62
globulin, sex hormone binding 45
gold-198 133
gonadotrophin and hormone therapy 160
– human chorionic 56
granulomatous prostatitis 68
grey scale sonogram 80
growth fraction 36
– hormone 48
– kinetics 29
– rate 29
gynaecomastia 177

histological grading 62
– –, Broder's 62
– –, Gleason's 62
– –, lymph node metastases 64, 125
– –, prognosis 128, 144
– –, treatment policy 133
– –, tumour state 125, 114, 115
honvan 160
hormonal status 47
hormones, see androgens
–, – anti-androgens
–, – oestrogens
–, – prednisone
–, – prednimustine
–, – progesterones
hormone sensitivity, normal gland 21
– –, neoplastic gland 154f
– therapy, see endocrine therapy
hydroxyproline excretion 115
hydroxyurea 149, 168
hyperplasia, see benign hyperplasia
hypertrophy, see benign hyperplasia
hypophysectomy, see pituitary ablation
hypoxia in tumors 148
hypoxic cell sensitizers 149

impotence after radiotherapy 143
– after surgery 144
incidence 2f, 173
– Caucasian 45
– familial 6
– international 5
– Japanese 6, 45
– Non-Whites 5, 7
– racial 179
– Whites 5, 7
incidental carcinoma, pathology 64
indium bleomycin 108
infection, venereal 8
–, viral 8
interferon 34
intermitotic time 29
interstitital irradiation 132
– –, survival rates 133, 134, 181
intraduct carcinoma 69
intravenous urography 76
– –, prognosis 145
invasion, nuclei 63
– perineural spaces 64
– prostatic capsule 66
iodine-125 128, 181
iridium-192 133
irradiation volume 141
isotope scans, see radionuclide scanning

kinetics 29

labelling index 31
latent cancer 2, 45
– –, management 157
liver disease 8
localized disease, therapeutic trial 181
– –, management 132, 158
lymphadenectomy 126

lymph node metastases 124
– confirmed histologically 126, 139
– histological grade 64, 125, 127
– incidence 103
– management 138
– and prognosis 106
– radiology 100
– site distribution 125, 139
– and tumour stage 125, 139
lymphography, accuracy 98, 139
– diagnostic strategy 94
– limitations 97
– results by T stage 104
– technique 98f
– vs lymphadenectomy 126
lymphoscintigraphy 109
luteinising hormone 45

marital status 8
markers, tumour 44
medroxyprogesterone acetate 160, 163
megestrol acetate 160
melphalan 149, 168
metaplastic changes 21, 32
– –, squamous 67
metastatic disease and growth hormone 48
– –, incidence by T stage 176
– –, management 159
methyl-CCNU 155, 168
misonidazole 149
mitosis labelled 29
mitotic index 29
– rate 29
morbidity from chemotherapy 154, 177
– from prostatic cancer 177
– from radiotherapy 143
– from surgery 128
mortality data 2
– rates 174
mucinous carcinoma 71
– secretion, sulphated sialo-mucin 62

National Prostatic Cancer Project 166
needle biopsy 121
neutron irradiation 149
nitrogen mustard 149
nitrosamines 154
nuclear morphometry, see computerised

occult carcinoma, management 174, 175, 178
– –, pathology 67
occupational risks 12, 13
oestradiol-17β 45, 50
oestrogen, radioactive labelled 108
– receptors 50
– – and radionuclide scanning 108
– therapy 44, 147, 154f
– – complications 129
orchiectomy 129, 154
– MRC trial 180

pathological classification 60
perineural infiltration 61
peripheral zone 22
phases – cell cycle 39
phenylalanine mustard, see melphalan
phosphatases, see acid and alkaline phosphatase
phosphorus-32 132
pituitary ablation 129, 160
polyamines in plasma 51
– in urine 54
population screening 13
potential doubling time 30
prednimustine 155, 166
prednisone 169
premalignant changes 44
Premarin 159
pre-operative radiotherapy 148
presenting features 176
primate prostate 21
procarbazine 156, 166, 167
progestogens 160
prognosis, age 176
–, histological grade 144, 145
–, M stage 116, 181
–, N stage 106, 181
–, T stage 140, 145
–, urography 145
prolactin 45
proliferating cells 29
prostatectomy 150
–, complications 128
–, radical 127, 157
–, survival rates 128, 181
prostatic ducts 20
prostatic growth 50
– –, regulation 50
– –, stimulation 50
– massage smears 14
– tumours, experimental 34
prostatitis 25
–, granulomatous 68
–, radiology 94
–, ultrasound diagnosis 86
prostatography 77, 80
Provera 159

radiocolloids 132
radiology 76f
–, diagnostic strategy 94
radionuclide scanning 77, 79
radiotherapy, complications 142
–, interstitial 132f
–, extended field 141
–, external beam 135f
–, small field 142
–, survival rates 181, 135f
receptors, androgen 38, 50
–, oestrogen 50
rectal carcinoma 68
– injury, postradiation 143
– ultrasound probe 83
religion 9
–, Jews 9
–, Mormons 9
–, Seventh day adventists 9
response to treatment, bone scan 115
– clinical assessment 165
– histology 92
– radiology 136

salivary gland steroids 48
scanner, rectilinear 111
–, multidetector 111
screening 13, 179
– acid phosphatase 14
– ultrasound 86
self-examination 175
seminal vesiculography 77, 79
sex hormone-binding globulin 45
sexual behaviour 8, 50
site of origin 25
size of prostate, calculation 78
– –, computed tomography 90, 92
– –, ultrasound 86
skeletal survey 125
small bowel injury 143
social class 10
spermidine 51
spermine 51
squamous cell carcinoma 71
– metaplasia 67
stage classification, American 157
–, UICC (TNM) 122f, 157
–, VACURG 157
stage correlations, acid phosphatase 125
– –, distribution at presentation 175
– –, histological grade 114
– –, investigation 125
– –, T & M categories 114, 125
– –, T & N categories 114, 106, 125
statistics, international 5
–, mortality 2
–, routine 1
steroid receptors 50
stilboestrol 154, 163, 164, 181
streptozotocin 166
strontium-85 112
– 87m 112
surgical management 127
survival rate by age 176
–, prostatectomy 128, 176
–, radiotherapy
– –, external beam 135f
– –, interstitial 132f
– – for Scotland 176

Tace 160
tantalum-182 133
technetium pyrophosphate 110
– methylenediphosphate 110
– ethanehydroxydiphosphonate 110
testesterone, effect on cell proliferation 38
–, peripheral zone epithelium 26
–, prostate growth 34, 38
–, plasma 45, 50, 129, 159, 182
thymidine labelling index 31
tobacco 11
tomochemistry 88
transitional cell carcinoma, bladder 69
– – –, prostatic ducts 69
– – –, urethra 69
– zone 24
transrectal biopsy 14
Tru-Cut biopsy 121
– needle 67
tumour grade, see histological grade
turnover time 30

ultrasonography 80f, 179
–, benign hyperplasia 84
–, perineal 82
–, suprapubic 80
–, transabdominal 80
–, transrectal 82
–, transurethral 82
ultrasound tomography 85
urethral cancer 69
urine cytology 14
urogenital sinus 20

VACURG 15, 154
–, trials 154f
venereal disease 8
venography 77, 78

vincristine 155, 168
vindesine 168
virus cytomegalus 8
– herpes 8
volume, irradiation, see irradiation volume
– prostatic, see size of prostate

xenografts 35
X-ray therapy 134f

yttrium-90 chloride 132
– seeds 129

zinc 14
– in normal prostate 21
– in secretory granules 25
zone, radioactive 79

Recent Results in Cancer Research

Sponsored by the Swiss League against Cancer. Editor in Chief: P. Rentchnick, Genève

For information about Vols. 1–9, please contact your bookseller of Springer-Verlag

10 NELSON, R. S.: Radioactive Phosphorus in the Diagnosis of Gastrointestinal Cancer.
11 FREEMAN, R. G. and J. M. KNOX: Treatment of Skin Cancer.
12 LYNCH, H. T.: Hereditary Factors in Carcinoma.
13 Tumours in Children, 2nd Edition. Edited by H. B. MARSDEN and J. K. STEWARD.
14 ODARTCHENKO, N.: Production Cellulaire Erythropoïétique.
15 SOKOLOFF, B.: Carcinoid and Serotonin.
16 JACOBS, M. L.: Malignant Lymphomas and Their Management.
17 Normal and Malignant Cell Growth. Edited by R. J. M. FRY, M. L. GRIEM, and W. H. KIRSTEN (Symposium).
18 ANGLESIO, E.: The Treatment of Hodgkin's Disease.
19 BANNASCH, P.: The Cytoplasm of Hepatocytes during Carcinogenesis. Electron- and Lightmicroscopical Investigations of the Nitrosomorpholineintoxicated Rat Liver.
20 Rubidomycin. A new Agent against Cancer. Edited by J. BERNARD, R. PAUL, M. BOIRON, C. JACQUILLAT, and R. MARAL.
21 Scientific Basis of Cancer Chemotherapy. Edited by G. MATHÉ (Symposium).
22 KOLDOVSKÝ, P.: Tumor Specific Transplantation Antigen.
23 FUCHS, W. A., J. W. DAVIDSON, and H. W. FISCHER: Lymphography in Cancer. With contributions by G. JANTET AND H. RÖSLER.
24 HAYWARD, J.: Hormones und Human Breast Cancer. An Account of 15 Years Study.
25 ROY-BURMAN, P.: Analogues of Nucleic Acid Components. Mechanisms of Action.
26 Tumors of the Liver. Edited by G. T. PACK and A. H. ISLAMI.
27 SZYMENDERA, J.: Bone Mineral Metabolism in Cancer.
28 MEEK, E. S.: Antitumour and Antiviral Substances of Natural Origin.
29 Aseptic Environments and Cancer Treatment. Edited by G. MATHÉ (Symposium).
30 Advances in the Treatment of Acute (Blastic) Leukemias. Edited by G. MATHÉ (Symposium).
31 DENOIX, P.: Treatment of Malignant Breast Tumors. Indications and Results.
32 NELSON, R. S.: Endoscopy in Gastric Cancer.
33 Experimental and Clinical Effects of L-Asparaginase. Edited by E. GRUNDMANN and H. F. OETTGEN (Symposium).
34 Chemistry and Biological Actions of 4-Nitroquinolin 1-Oxide. Edited by H. ENDO, T. ONO, and T. SUGIMURA.
35 PENN, I.: Malignant Tumors in Organ Transplant Recipients.
36 Current Concepts in the Management of Lymphoma and Leukemia. Edited by J. E. ULTMANN, M. L. GRIEM, W. H. KIRSTEN, and R. W. WISSLER (Symposium).
37 CHIAPPA, S., R. MUSUMECI, and C. USLENGHI: Endolymphatic Radiotherapy in Malignant Lymphomas. With contributions by G. BONADONNA, B. DAMASCELLI, G. FAVA, F. PIZZETTI, U. VERONESI.
38 KOLLER, P. C.: The Role of Chromosomes in Cancer Biology.
39 Current Problems in the Epidemiology of Cancer and Lymphomas. Edited by E. GRUNDMANN and H. TULINIUS (Symposium).
40 LANGLEY, F. A. and A. C. CROMPTON: Epithelial Abnormalities of the Cervix Uteri.
41 Tumours in a Tropical Country. A Survey of Uganda (1964–1968). Edited by A. C. TEMPLETON.
42 Breast Cancer: A Challenging Problem. Edited by M. L. GRIEM, E. V. JENSEN, J. E. ULTMANN, and R. W. WISSLER (Symposium).
43 Nomenclature, Methodology and Results of Clinical Trials in Acute Leukemias. Edited by G. MATHÉ, P. POUILLART, L. SCHWARZENBERG (Symposium).
44 Special Topics in Carcinogenesis. Edited by E. GRUNDMANN (Symposium).
45 KOLDOVSKÝ, P.: Carcinoembryonic Antigens.
46 Diagnosis and Therapy of Malignant Lymphoma. Edited by K. MUSSHOFF (Symposium).
47 Investigation and Stimulation of Immunity in Cancer Patients. Edited by G. MATHÉ and R. WEINER (Symposium).
48 Platinum Coordination Complexes in Cancer Chemotherapy. Edited by T. A. CONNORS and J. J. ROBERTS (Symposium).
49 Complications of Cancer Chemotherapy. Edited by G. MATHÉ and R. K. OLDHAM (Symposium).
50 Cancer Registry, Edited by E. GRUNDMANN and E. PEDERSEN (Symposium).
51 Gliomas. Current Concepts in Biology, Diagnosis and Therapy. Edited by J. HEKMATPANAH (Symposium).

52 The Ambivalence of Cytostatic Therapy. Edited by E. GRUNDMANN and R. GROSS (Symposium).
53 A. CLARYSSE, Y. KENIS, and G. MATHÉ: Cancer Chemotherapy.
54 Malignant Bone Tumors. Edited by E. GRUNDMANN.
55 MATHÉ, G.: Cancer Active Immunotherapy, Immunoprophylaxis, and Immunorestoration.
56 Lymphocytes, Macrophages, and Cancer. Edited by G. MATHÉ, I. FLORENTIN, and M.-C. SIMMLER (Symposium).
57 Breast Cancer: A Multidisciplinary Approach. Edited by G. ST. ARNEAULT, P. BAND, and L. ISRAËL (Symposium).
58 B. S. SCHOENBERG: Multiple Primary Malignant Neoplasms.
59 Selective Heat Sensitivity of Cancer Cells. Edited by A. ROSSI-FANELLI, R. CAVALIERE, B. MONDOVI, and G. MORICCA.
60 Tumors of the Male Genital System. Edited by E. GRUNDMANN and W. VAHLENSIECK (Symposium).
61 D. METCALF: Hemopoietic Colonies.
62 Tactics and Strategy in Cancer Treatment. Edited by G. MATHÉ (Symposium).
63 Antitumor Antibiotics. Edited by S. K. CARTER, H. UMEZAWA, J. DOUROS, and Y. SAKURAI (Symposium).
64 Lymphoid Neoplasias I: Classification, Categorization, Natural History.
65 Lymphoid Neoplasias II: Clinical and Therapeutic Aspects.
Lymphoid Neoplasias I & II. Proceedings of the 1977 CNRS-EORTC International Colloquium. Editors: G. MATHÉ, M. SELIGMANN, M. TUBIANA. Devided into two volumes.
66 Carcinogenic Hormones. Edited by C. H. LINGEMAN.
67/68 Adjuvant Therapies and Markers of Post-Surgical Minimal Residual Disease I & II. Proceedings of the 1978 Annual Plenary Meeting of the EORTC. Editors: G. BONADONNA, G. MATHÉ, S. E. SALMON. Divided into two volumes.
67 Markers and General Problems of Cancer Adjuvant Therapies.
68 Adjuvant Therapies of the Various Primary Tumors.
69 Strategies in Clinical Hematology. Edited by R. GROSS and K.-P. HELLRIEGEL.
70 New Anticancer Drugs. Edited by S. K. CARTER
71 Endocrine Treatment of Breast Cancer. Edited by B. HENNINGSEN, F. LINDER, C. STREICHELE.
72 CAWLEY, J. C., BURNS, G. F., HAYHOE, F. G. J.: Hairy-Cell Leukaemia.
73 Thyroid Cancer. Edited by W. DUNCAN.
74 Cancer Chemo- and Immunopharmacology. 1. Chemopharmacology. Edited by G. MATHÉ and F. M. MUGGIA.
75 Cancer Chemo- and Immunopharmacology. 2. Immunopharmacology, Relations and General Problems. Edited by G. MATHÉ and F. M. MUGGIA.
76 New Drugs in Cancer Chemotherapy. Edited by S. K. CARTER, Y. SAKURAI, H. UMEZAWA
77 K. STANLEY, J. STJERNSWÄRD, M. ISLEY: The Conduct of a Cooperative Clinical Trial.
78 Prostate Cancer. Edited by W. DUNCAN.

MIX
Papier aus verantwortungsvollen Quellen
Paper from responsible sources
FSC® C105338
FSC
www.fsc.org

If you have any concerns about our products,
you can contact us on
ProductSafety@springernature.com

In case Publisher is established outside the EU,
the EU authorized representative is:
Springer Nature Customer Service Center GmbH
Europaplatz 3, 69115 Heidelberg, Germany

Printed by Libri Plureos GmbH
in Hamburg, Germany